touches your heart

Jerry

7/8/24 .

Embracing My Scars

EMBRACING MY SCARS

A journey of hope in the face of adversity

JERRY MORRISSEY

Embracing My Scars
First published in Australia
Copyright © Jerry Morrissey 2024

Extracts from the following case report are reprinted in this book: N Tanner and M Pickford, 'Preliminary report: intratumoral ligation as a salvage procedure for the management of life-threatening arteriovenous malformations', *British Journal of Plastic Surgery*, 1993, 46(8):694–702, doi: 10.1016/0007-1226(93)90202-m

Typeset and cover design by BookPOD

ISBN: 978-1-7636391-0-2 (pbk) eISBN: 978-1-7636391-1-9 (e-book)

NATIONAL LIBRARY OF AUSTRALIA

A catalogue record for this book is available from the National Library of Australia

Contents

Triumph over the Darkness

This story has taken me over thirty years to write. Some people said it would be cathartic. Truthfully, recounting the chapters of my life has compelled me to relive some harrowing experiences that part of me would rather forget.

Throughout the process, even when my conscious mind seemed settled, my subconscious would wake me in the dead of night from the nightmares that haunted me – visions of my mother enduring horrific brutality at the hands of my father and the chilling sensation of almost bleeding to death on multiple occasions. The profound realisation that your life is slipping away from you and there's nothing you can do about it. I wouldn't wish it on anyone.

This is a story that touches the depths of the human condition – violence, fear, morality and death. It's also a story about love and triumphing over negativity. The truth is, I thought no one would ever love me with my disfigured face and mangled, scarred body. But I am here to tell you that anything is possible. I am living proof of that.

The World Health Organization estimates that over 700,000 people take their own life each year – that's one person every forty seconds. For each suicide, there are an estimated twenty suicide attempts. I was one of those statistics. At eighteen years of age, I wanted to die. I wrestled with deep, dark suicidal thoughts and I attempted suicide in my final year at boarding school.

I survived and went on to face some monumental challenges – mental and physical – over the next few years. At one point, in reference to an operation I faced, a doctor described it as 'temporarily killing Jerry … then starting him back up again'. Another described it as 'a post-mortem on a living body'. Again I survived. However, due to a post-operative stroke, I was trapped in my body, paralysed on the right-hand side and unable to see or speak. It took months of rehabilitation to function as a normal human being again.

In this book, I describe firsthand how your greatest battles are won or lost in your mind. For me, it was a challenge both internally and externally to reach a stage where I was comfortable in my own skin – but I am here today as testament to the fact that you can triumph over your own internal darkness.

If this story prevents only one person from taking their own life or helps them out of a dark place to enjoy the best life they can, then the pain I experienced in this life and in writing this book will have been worth it.

PART 1

BORN IN A WAR ZONE

CHAPTER 1

Life in the Drum

No matter where you grow up or what you may experience, it is possible to escape the circumstances you were born into and create a better life for yourself. My life is just one example of that.

As a small boy growing up in Drumchapel on the outskirts of Glasgow, I was exposed to the light and shade of Glaswegian life in the 1960s and '70s. From poverty and domestic violence to community and a shared sense of care, the Drum – as we locals called it – offered plenty of both.

Drumchapel was one of the 'big four' council-owned housing estates – along with Easterhouse, Castlemilk and Greater Pollok – built after the Second World War to cater for the thousands of slum-dwellers from inner city Glasgow.

Comedian Billy Connolly's family was among those shipped out to the new housing schemes. He referred to the Drum as a 'desert wi' windaes' and he wasn't wrong. It was as if the Drum was monochrome, with long bleak-looking rows of cheaply made tenement blocks. It was high-density living, yet it was in a beautiful area west of Glasgow. To the north was a woodland that in springtime was carpeted with bluebells, and, beyond that, a golf course and the district of Bearsden and Milngavie, one of the most affluent areas in the UK, full of old Victorian houses.

Because of this backdrop, the Drum could look quite beautiful, so the council's intent made sense. But in practice, it didn't have any infrastructure or amenities, especially when it was first established, which caused all kinds of social problems.

I was around four years of age when we moved there. Before that we lived in Springburn, but I don't remember those early years. My birth certificate tells me I was born at Oakbank Hospital in Possilpark, near where my granny lived, but my first memories are of starting primary school in Drumchapel.

We lived on Summerhill Road in a three-storey tenement block known as a 'close' with six other families in separate apartments. If someone raised their voice, everyone in the building could hear it as the walls were so flimsy. There was a common ground-floor entrance that provided access to the staircase, which went up three flights with an apartment on either side on each floor.

Our apartment was on the top floor on the right-hand side of the staircase, and it had two small bedrooms. My parents had one and I had the other. My sister, Sharon, didn't come along until later so, in those early years, I had the bedroom to myself. In our apartment we had a black-and-white television, a record player and a radio, which in the colder weather occupied much of my time. The only heating was an electric heater with one bar, which meant that in winter, even just a few feet away from the heater, it was freezing cold. In the morning the bedroom windows would be iced up and you could lie in bed and breathe out in a misty cloud, which wasn't much incentive to get up and get ready for school.

You got to know your neighbours pretty well in those cramped conditions and my mother was friends with all of them. Nobody had a car, so, if you wanted to go anywhere, you had to catch a bus or walk. Despite the poverty, it felt like we were all in it together. There was a mutual reliance and a strong sense of community, with everyone looking out for each other, so you were never actually lonely in the Drum.

Many of the local people worked at the nearby shipyards at Clydebank. There were a number of ships being built at any one time, and it was a hive of activity. The men were welders, caulkers, platers, burners, joiners, engineers and electricians. They worked long hours and got paid on a Friday, at which point they would head straight to the pub. Celtic and Rangers were the two big premiership-side football clubs based in Glasgow and everybody was into football (soccer), so, depending on who they supported, they'd either head to the Celtic pub or the Rangers pub, both of which would be heaving for the whole weekend.

Gangs and gang warfare provided the backdrop for life in the Drum, though I, of course, was too young to be involved in any of that. I knew it was there but it didn't really affect my life. Drinking and domestic violence were rife, and the neighbours all had their own issues and personal battles. We would hear yelling and screaming and banging from the tenements as us kids played outside, but we would just focus on each other and ignore the escalating noise – it was all a normal part of growing up in the Drum and we knew no different.

It was an era before the digital age and before computer games, so in summer we were outside exploring the Bluebell Woods. There were little burns, or streams, and fields with grazing cattle nearby. I would play with the Connelly kids, who lived in the close next door, and some other neighbourhood kids. We would roam the woods, climb the trees, make little dens and pick the wild rhubarb, which we would bring home and feast on, raw and dipped in sugar. Show jumping must have been popular at the time too, because we made an obstacle course with an old oil drum as a jump, and I ended up slicing my calf open on it. I ran home, blood pouring down my leg. Mum carted me off to hospital to have butterfly strips applied to seal up the wound – the scar remains to this day.

If we weren't in the woods, we were playing out the back of the tenement or on the road. There was a big communal, rectangular, grassed garden space where the washing lines were. We'd play our obstacle course game there too with large stainless steel rubbish bins, and we'd play football and a little game called Kerby, which involved throwing a ball across the road at the kerb and catching it when it bounced back to you to score a point. On 5 November it was bonfire night, and we spent the two weeks prior gathering everything we could from the neighbourhood bins, as well as branches from the woods, to burn in a bonfire out the back of the close.

My father, Big Jerry, was older than my mother. He'd been in the British Army, so he'd seen a bit of life. My mum, Margaret, was just nineteen when they met. Big Jerry was twenty-five, charming and not a bad-looking guy, with dark wavy hair and a moustache. Mum was one of seven kids and hadn't had a great life growing up. Her parents split up and her mother, my granny, had remarried a horrible guy, Charlie, who beat my granny up. Mum just wanted to get away, and Big Jerry presented that opportunity.

He was an Irish Catholic and my mother was a Scottish Protestant, which was a big deal in those days on the west coast of Scotland. But they married anyway on 14 November 1961, and I was born in 1964.

Because Big Jerry was Catholic, I was sent to St Pius – the local Catholic primary school in the Drum. I was the first person on Mum's side of the family to be sent to a Catholic school. In

Scotland, particularly on the west coast, the whole Catholic/ Protestant thing was a nightmare – like a war zone, same as in Northern Ireland. It wasn't until years later I realised what that religious dynamic meant. You would be asked what school you'd attended and were very often judged or ignored as soon as the word 'Saint…' came out of your mouth.

Big Jerry was a bus driver, and he got paid on a Friday and went straight to the pub like all the other local men. He drank and gambled away all his earnings, and there would be no money left for the rest of the week. Then he would stagger up the road home after consuming vast amounts of alcohol.

I would be on the lookout for him from the window of our top-floor flat. One Friday evening, I was hanging out the window to check if I could see him coming, because I knew the madness would start and I wanted to warn Mum. I stretched my body as far as I could out the window to get a better view and as I turned my head this way and that, trying to cover all angles, I lost my balance and started to fall. It was a good thirty-metre drop to the concrete outside the apartment, and, in my panic not to launch out the window, I managed to twist and turn in the air like a cat and fall back into the apartment instead. Aiming to land on all fours, instead I landed headfirst on the record player and split my head open.

Blood poured in rivulets down my face and neck. Mum hurriedly wrapped a tea towel around my head to soak up the blood, then called an ambulance. I was taken to the hospital to be stitched up. Another scar that remains to this day. At least it saved my mother from one of Big Jerry's savage beatings, but I couldn't pull something like that every time he went to the pub.

You could never tell when the madness was going to start.

It depended on how long he was in the pub, how drunk he was when he came back and what mood he was in. We were always anticipating how he would be. Would it be a good mood or a bad mood today? You couldn't predict it, though if Celtic got beaten, he would be so pissed off that we knew he'd take it out on Mum, so we always kept an eye on the football scores. But the truth was, he could always find something to set him off, and it was always Mum's fault. Nothing she could do was ever good enough for him, and he'd feel compelled to dish out a beating to show her what was what. And so the cycle of domestic violence would repeat itself like a never-ending nightmare…

One night, I awoke to hear my mother screaming for help in the early hours of the morning. 'No, no, please no…' she begged, sobbing and choking on her tears. There was a loud banging and smacking sound as he hit her again. She begged him to stop, pleading for her life, shrieking in pain. I couldn't stop shaking and crying as I listened, wrapped in my thick blankets, hiding under the covers. There was nothing I could do to help her, and the guilt I felt was visceral. He told me to stay in my room and not come out under any circumstances, and I was way too afraid to defy him. I was only a small boy – what could I do? He was a big man – people called him Big Jerry for a reason. He was a trained soldier, and violence was part of his nature.

Things quietened down for a bit and I started to calm down slightly, then it started up again cyclically until the wee small hours of the morning when Big Jerry passed out. It happened during the day sometimes as well, but it always seemed worse at night – everything became amplified in the darkness. To hear my mum pleading for her life – it's a terror I will never forget.

The next day she was battered and bruised, and her eyes

were puffy from the tears. But whatever she felt emotionally, she kept to herself. She would be quiet for a few days … subdued, sad … but still put a smile on her face to go to her job at the local supermarket. She never wanted anyone to see her misery. And Big Jerry would just carry on as if everything was normal. It was a scene that played out regularly. Sometimes he would apologise; more often than not, he wouldn't.

Sometimes he'd send me to get something from the shop, but I knew it was just a ploy to get me out of the house so he could start hitting my mum. Other times he was quite happy to slap and punch her right there in front of me.

It was better on days when he'd get home and just start playing records loudly – Simon & Garfunkel's *Bridge Over Troubled Water* and the Glaswegian country singer Sydney Devine. I would stay out of his way, but there was still this constant feeling of being on edge, wondering when the madness would begin again.

The mere sight of Big Jerry's piercing gaze ignited a storm of fear within me. My heart would race uncontrollably, my body trembling in dread of his next violent outburst. I felt myself shrinking inward, withdrawing into a shell of isolation.

I began to internalise everything. I learned to withdraw into myself. Powerless and confused, I struggled to grasp a true sense of reality, lost in a perpetual state of anxiety that clouded every moment of my young life.

Hopelessness became my constant companion, as I saw no end to the nightmare that played out on repeat, each day blending into the next with no respite. My body remained on high alert, aching for safety that never came.

CHAPTER 2

A Game of Cat and Mouse

Mum tried leaving him a few times in the late '60s and we went to stay with my granny in Possilpark. Inevitably, though, Big Jerry would turn up on Granny's doorstep and sweet-talk Mum into coming back. He'd use that charm of his. No one would ever have believed what he was really like behind closed doors. If you spoke to his work colleagues – the other bus drivers he enjoyed a few pints or betting on the horses with – in that macho male culture, they would say he was always smiling, and everyone thought he was a top guy. They had no idea he had such a dark side … but we knew only too well.

On one occasion when we were staying at Granny's – it must have been 1969 – he turned up to woo Mum back with a new approach. 'Come back, come back,' he said. 'We'll have another baby and everything will be alright.' And back we went, into the fray…

Mum was soon pregnant, but it didn't change a thing – if anything it made him worse. She would pick me up from school and we'd walk back to the close on Summerhill Road. If Big Jerry had worked the early shift on the buses, he'd be home about lunchtime, waiting for us on the landing outside our apartment. As we climbed the stairs, we'd see him standing there, with a sick, twisted smile on his face – the one that let you know he held all the cards as to whether you were going to be safe or not. Sometimes he would let us through into the apartment but other times he'd wait until Mum was about to step onto the landing and he'd kick her down the stairs, smiling all the while, just because he could. What kind of monster kicks a pregnant woman down the stairs?

My sister, Sharon, was born in 1970. Soon afterwards, my mother was admitted to a psychiatric hospital, suffering from a complete mental breakdown, and put on medication. No surprises there. Sharon and I were packed off to go and stay with Granny. After Mum was discharged from the hospital some weeks later, we returned to Drumchapel and the pattern of domestic violence resumed.

In the end, two incidents occurred that finally made her decide to leave for good. The first took place at home while I was in the lounge, playing *Top of the Pops* records on the turntable. They were arguing loudly in the kitchen. The next thing I knew, she was screaming blue murder and racing into the lounge to get away. I found out later he'd thrown a massive chip pan full of hot oil right at her. Somehow, it had missed her and hit the wall. He chased her into the lounge room, red-faced and panting as he pinned her down on the settee right next to where I was sitting and put his big hands around her throat. She was choking right in front of my eyes and I couldn't stop myself that time. I launched myself at him and tried to pull him off her. Throwing his arm back violently, I went flying across the room. That's when Mum began pleading with him on my behalf, somehow managing to defuse the situation and calm him down long enough to get me out of the house.

Around this time I had begun wetting the bed every night. At the age of nine, the burden of bed-wetting inflicted deep emotional wounds on me. I carried an overwhelming sense of responsibility, constantly blaming myself for the turmoil at home. Night after night, I endured a toxic blend of fear and guilt, fully aware of the inevitable consequences of my bed-wetting and the explosive anger it triggered in Big Jerry. His violent reactions turned my bed-wetting into a closely guarded secret, shared only between my mother and me.

Mornings became a silent battlefield, where my unspoken exchanges with my mother (we couldn't risk Big Jerry overhearing us) were filled with nods that determined whether my night had been dry or soaked. If it was the latter, my mother would quietly remove my soiled bed sheets and pyjamas, offering solace through her gentle actions. She would open my bedroom window to reduce the nauseating stench of urine. The persistent dampness on my body led to a raw, painful rash on my thighs and genitals that would sometimes bleed – a physical manifestation of my hidden shame and embarrassment. Each day, before facing the world at school, I endured the stinging ritual of washing and soothing my inflamed skin with a talc-based body powder.

Eventually, Mum took me to the doctor. He asked a little about our home environment and she told him the truth. He told her in no uncertain terms to get out of there: 'Because if you don't, your son is going to suffer from severe mental health or behavioural problems down the track.'

It was the final straw. The next day, Mum waited until Big Jerry went to work, then threw our belongings – whatever we could carry – into polythene bags. She told me and Sharon, who was two by then, that we were leaving.

We caught a bus and then another bus to Possilpark. It was only about ten kilometres away (as the crow flies), but at the time it felt like hours of being on the road. I felt sick – whether from motion or emotion, I'm not sure. 'Stop the bus, stop the bus!' Mum called out to the driver. 'My son's going to throw up!' I got off the bus just in time and vomited into the gutter. We walked the final kilometre or two to Granny's house, where Mum announced she had left Big Jerry for good this time. Granny said we could stay for as long as it took for the emergency system (which provided safe emergency shelter for women and children escaping domestic violence) to find somewhere for us to live.

The next Sunday, Mum took Sharon and me down to the Barras, a historic market in the East End of Glasgow. Since we'd left most of our belongings behind in the Drum, she wanted to buy some bits and pieces for the council flat we were hoping would soon be allocated. We were perusing the stalls full of furniture, clothes, jewellery, ornaments, paintings and toys when she spotted him across the market. Big Jerry was surveying the scene, scanning the crowds, looking for us. Perhaps he'd followed us all the way from Granny's. Mum quickly pulled us under the nearest stall table, and we huddled together, holding our breath behind the hanging tablecloth as he passed by.

That's how it was … we never felt safe. He was always looking for us. I don't know if he really wanted us back or if he just wanted to feel like he controlled us. Either way, it was a game of cat and mouse that left us all in a constant state of anxiety. We were always looking over our shoulders and expecting the worst.

I've often wondered whether Big Jerry was mad or just bad … but he knew what he was doing. He planned it all out so he was in control, and, to me, that suggests he was just bad. It's hard to know why he was the way he was, because his parents seemed nice enough when we visited them in Dublin. And there wasn't a hint of Big Jerry's brutal behaviour on the several occasions we went to visit them. We'd catch the ferry from Stranraer to Belfast, hire a car and drive across the border down to Dublin. As we'd go through the checkpoint at the border, soldiers in combat gear would have their guns trained on us. Big Jerry's mum and dad lived in Thomas Street in central Dublin, near the Guinness Factory. I always felt really comfortable in their home and only have positive memories of them.

Later, my mother speculated whether Big Jerry was working for the IRA. The Irish Republican Army was a paramilitary organisation that sought the end of British rule in Northern Ireland and reunification with the south. Some considered them to be terrorists, while others saw them as freedom fighters. Either way, it was odd that we caught the ferry to Northern Ireland when we could have gone straight to Dublin. Was Big Jerry a secret gun runner posing as a family man? Who knows…

Soon enough the council found us an apartment in Springburn, just to the east of Possilpark, and I started school nearby. The ground-floor flat was a 'single-end' – a Glaswegian term for a one-room apartment. The bedroom, kitchen, living room, bathroom and toilet were all in the one room. It was in a long, narrow tenement building with one main entrance and a long central hallway with lots of single-end rooms off it.

Soon after we settled in, predictably, Big Jerry came looking for us. And then a devastating scenario began to play out, again and again. He'd pitch up at Granny's first and look for movements in and out of her house, because he knew we'd be there visiting a couple of times a week. If he didn't find us there, he'd phone up all the schools in the area that started with 'Saint', since he knew I went to a Catholic school – St Pius, St Aloysius, St Cuthbert. He'd take a scattergun approach, phoning all the schools in the area and saying he had a message for his son. Once he'd confirmed which school I attended, he'd hide in the bushes outside the school gates and wait for all the kids to come out at the end of the school day. Then he'd follow me home but at a distance so I didn't know he was there.

Once I'd gone inside, he'd knock and Mum would answer the door. He'd start hollering at her, threatening her, and end up bashing her yet again, while Sharon and I hid inside. Then he would disappear, and Mum would say it wasn't safe there anymore now that he knew where we were. So, we would pack our stuff and head back to Granny's house until we could get emergency accommodation and somewhere else to live.

Maybe he was just playing a daft game – once he found us, he knew we would have to leave, and the cycle would start again.

After Springburn, we moved to an apartment in Possilpark and then it was on to Maryhill – another single-end. I remember that place because of the multicoloured streamers that hung down in front of the toilet for some element of privacy since there was no door. We weren't there for long before we were told the building was going to be demolished, so it was back to Granny's for another stint.

Whenever we stayed with Granny, it was just as bad as being at home with Big Jerry, since her second husband, Charlie, was also a violent drunk. There was this little gas heater that you fed coins in to keep the heating on. Charlie would sit in front of it, hogging the warmth and scaring everyone. Granny's place was also in a tenement and not much bigger than our place in the Drum, though it was a bit more solid. There were only two rooms – we called them 'the big room' and 'the wee room' – plus a kitchen and toilet.

You might question how Granny ended up marrying someone like Charlie, but she had been told her first husband (Mum's father) was killed fighting in the Second World War. He was a paratrooper in the Parachute Regiment and had been involved in the famous Battle of Arnhem. However, he didn't die in the battle, as she had been told. He was captured and became a prisoner of war for many years. When he was finally released, Granny had already met Charlie and married him. I wish we'd had the chance to get to know my real grandfather.

Granny had her other kids and grandkids staying over often, in addition to us. Rose-Ann, Mum's younger sister, was there, and she had two kids about Sharon's age. Then there was Mum's youngest brother, Matthew, who was a teenager and still living at home. Since there were only two rooms, we'd sleep three or four to a bed or on the couch in the living room.

Charlie was a Protestant and a big follower of the Rangers, and all of his sons, my uncles, followed them too. Because I went to a Catholic school, I was the odd one out, so it was never great for me at Granny's house.

Charlie would get drunk on a Friday night. It was my job to look out the window in the wee room to see when he was coming home. It was the same scenario as in the Drum – though this time I kept watch from the ground floor. We would see Charlie staggering up the road, steaming drunk, often with a chicken curry in his hand. His favourite drinking hole was the Rock Tavern, about half a kilometre from Granny's house. Granny would shout, 'He's coming,' and us kids would climb onto the settee and dive out the window to get away. There was a little square nearby where we'd hang out and watch the house from a distance, waiting until things calmed down a bit.

If things got really bad, Granny would tell us to run to the phone box, which was half a kilometre away on Possil Road, and call the police. The cops would come and take Charlie away. They'd lock him up in jail for thirty days for assault and battery, being drunk and disorderly, or both. That was always a relief – thirty days of respite – and it meant we could stay with Granny a bit longer.

One evening it wasn't Charlie I saw coming up the road, but Big Jerry. I spotted him when he was about 150 metres away. As soon as I was sure it was him and not Charlie, I yelled out to Mum and Granny, 'He's coming up the road but it's no' Charlie – it's ma da!'

My granny went into what can only be described as Operation Lockdown, locking all the windows and doors and making sure the chain was across on the front door. All us kids were moved into the living room area. When Big Jerry arrived, he started banging on the door.

'I know yer in there – open this effing door before I smash it in!'

He started kicking the front door in, and this rhythmic banging repeated itself for a few minutes. Then things grew quiet, but it was the calm before the storm. *Bang, smash, crash!* Big Jerry was breaking the windows in the wee room and climbing into the house. Granny, Mum, Sharon and I flew across the flat and climbed over the settee and out the back window. Legging it as fast as we could down to the phone box, we called the police who arrived quickly – after all, it was a common occurrence at Granny's house – and Big Jerry was taken away. We didn't see him for the next thirty days.

He insisted on seeing me, though, whenever we were staying at Granny's. He didn't want to know about Sharon – I don't know why – but he would take me to the football to see Celtic play. The last time I ever saw him was on one of those afternoons. I was twelve years old.

Big Jerry disappeared without a word.

He sold the furniture, cleared out the bank accounts and took off back to Ireland. He left us with nothing. We also found out later he'd taken a woman, posing as my mum, with him to the bank to close the accounts. We don't know who she was – probably a drinking buddy he'd lured in with the promise of a few free drinks.

Charlie must have been in jail because we stayed with my granny for quite some time, and I started at another school nearby, St Cuthberts, which was just around the corner in Possilpark. Mum had applied for another council flat and this time it was back to the Drum, to a close on Carolside Drive. The apartment was much the same size as the one on Summerhill Road, but we had a little verandah next to the living room.

I was paranoid Big Jerry would turn up there as well since he always seemed to find us, and we didn't know at this point that he was never going to return. I was fully expecting him to knock the door down and smash the windows, so I concocted a plan – I would make a house alarm that would alert us to any unexpected arrivals.

I had a small transistor radio – one of those plastic ones about the size of an iPhone – with an amplifier in it as well as capacitors and resistors. Stripping it apart, I pulled out the battery and amplifier to create an electrical circuit and used the plastic exterior unit to hold it all together, then I fixed it to the wall beside the door with duct tape. I affixed a piece of string to the door with the other end going into an eye socket in the plastic case of the radio, so if somebody opened the door, the alarm would go off.

It provided me with some small level of comfort, although, in the end, we never did see or hear from Big Jerry again. However, the damage he had caused was irreversible. Even as I started secondary school, memories of his unsettling behaviour – like following me home and hiding in bushes – lingered, leaving me with a persistent feeling of unease. I could never fully shake off the sense of vulnerability and danger.

It wasn't until many years later we heard what had become of Big Jerry when a woman from Ireland contacted me claiming she was my half-sister … but that's a story for a later chapter.

CHAPTER 3

Teen Spirit and My First Surgery

While we were still in Possilpark living with Granny, Mum had met a guy called George who lived just around the corner with his parents. She'd bump into him when we were out walking, and they'd stop and chat. It was obvious he was interested in her, even though she was ten years older than him. He probably thought they were the same age since she looked way younger than she was. Initially she told him we were her sister Rose-Ann's children, so she was clearly interested in him enough to lie about us. The truth must've come out at some stage, though, because once we moved to Carolside Drive – known as the posh end of Drumchapel because it was on the hill – George moved right on in. And Mum told us to tell the world he was our uncle. In those days, living together as an unmarried couple was frowned upon.

Mum was working in a local supermarket, and George got a job there too and became the manager. Sharon and I got on well with him. He was full of energy – in the army reserves as well as working full-time and into sports. We played tennis with him and did cross-country running as well.

It was a calm time for us after so many years of turmoil living with Big Jerry. In 1976, I started secondary school at St Pius in

Drumchapel while Sharon was at primary school. I'd walk up the hill to school and back down again after school until I got a bike when I was slightly older. We bought it down at the Barras. It was a second-hand racing bike and too big for me, but, because it was cheap, Mum said I'd grow into it when I got bigger. It should have been light since it was a racing bike, but this thing was cobbled together from different parts and it was heavy. One time I had an accident – I was coming down the hill and I couldn't stop in time. I came down the path and into Carolside Drive and went over the handlebars. No broken bones, though maybe some bruised pride, but I did learn not to go so fast on the hill.

I was clearly a motivated lad from a young age, as I had two paper rounds in high school. One on a Sunday morning was a massive round involving a few hundred newspapers with the Sunday supplement. I walked from Carolside Drive to Peel Glen, which was a couple of kilometres, to pick up the papers at the pick-up point at 6am. Then carrying them in two huge canvas bags, I walked back to Carolside Drive to start delivering. My round extended a further three kilometres in the other direction. Three hours after I delivered the papers, I'd go around the same route again to get my money from the delivery customers. From Monday to Saturday I had another smaller round. I was working seven days a week delivering the papers as well as going to school.

I discovered I had a talent for some extracurricular activities at high school too. I learned chess quickly and played for the school chess team. Later, we reached the final of the UK's *Sunday Times* Chess Championships. To get to the final, we beat the likes of top fee-paying independent schools like Edinburgh's George Heriot's. In the Scottish final, we lost by a mere half-point against top plush school Stewart's Melville College, also from Edinburgh.

I also played for the school table tennis team and reached the semi-final of the Scottish Schools Championships. So, despite the horrendous years of my childhood with Big Jerry and the Drum, I somehow managed to focus and apply myself.

Playing chess became a refuge from the violence I had witnessed, offering a stark contrast in its quiet and orderly setting. Chess provided a sense of control and tranquillity that was sorely lacking at home in my earliest years. The strategic nature of chess demanded intense concentration, forcing me to immerse myself completely in the intricacies of each move and anticipate my opponent's strategies. This mental challenge required me to block out all other distractions, including the chaos of my home life. Chess became a form of escapism, as I found solace in the structured and focused world of the game. It was a rare space where I could experience a sense of calmness and clarity.

My brother, Paul, was born in those years in Drumchapel too. I was already a teenager, but it was nice to have another small sibling and for Mum and George to have a baby together – it gave a real sense of family to our lives. Even as a baby, I remember Paul being fascinated by the Moon. I would hold him up and say, 'Can you see the man on the Moon?' and he would just stare at it for ages. It was something we shared together – I did it for years with him until he was too big to hold.

$\sim$

Life was pretty stable until I turned fourteen. That's when life got tumultuous again but in a very different kind of way. I had developed this throbbing pain in my gum and some swelling. Mum gave me some painkillers, which seemed to help – the swelling subsided and the pain went away. A few months later, it reoccurred. Again, I took painkillers and it disappeared. But a year after the first bout, it came back, this time with some external swelling and a pulse in my ears when I was trying to sleep.

Mum took me to the dentist as we both thought it was a rotten tooth needing a filling or extraction. That's what the dentist thought too – just a bad tooth. He was getting ready to remove it when an eagle-eyed dental student, who was simply there observing, suggested maybe it might be something more … and with hindsight, thank God he did. I might not be here today if the dentist had done the extraction.

The dentist x-rayed the gum and clearly didn't like what he saw. He referred me for an angiogram at Canniesburn Hospital, an internationally renowned hospital for plastic surgery, which just happened to be near Drumchapel. An angiogram or arteriogram is a scanning procedure that helps doctors detect abnormal blood vessels, clots and other problems, though of course I didn't know that at the time.

The doctor we saw there was a consultant plastic surgeon called Mr Moos. I told him about the pain and swelling coming and going over the previous twelve months, and that I'd also now noticed two small black objects in my left field of vision occasionally. After the angiogram, Mr Moos told us there might be a problem with the arteries and veins on the left-hand side of my face. He also told us they couldn't do anything for me – not him nor anyone else in Scotland – which, if I'd thought about it, might have indicated how serious the situation was since Canniesburn Hospital specialised in plastic and maxillofacial surgery, and there were a lot of key surgeons there.

He said it was because of the vascular nature of the thing and that there was a doctor in London, Professor Calnan, who was also a consultant plastic surgeon but worked alongside some top vascular surgeons at the Hammersmith Hospital in London. I had no idea what to think … there wasn't much going through my head, really. I was a teenager, after all. Just a daft kid with no concept of what was about to unfold. Plus, my face looked normal and symmetrical, with little evidence of the massive swelling that was to take control over the left side of my face.

On the upside, going to London for the first time seemed pretty exciting. In those days, you caught a train or a bus. The bus took about twelve hours overnight, while the train went during the day and took about six hours or so. London, the big capital! I had never ventured outside Drumchapel or even been out of Glasgow, except to go to Dublin to see Big Jerry's parents.

That trip to London was the first of many. I caught the bus on my own, and my aunt Agnes and uncle Jim met me at Euston Station and took me back to their house in Swiss Cottage. The next day they took me to the Hammersmith Hospital to meet with Professor Calnan, who looked at the results of the angiogram I'd had at Canniesburn and did a range of tests.

There were a good few months of investigations. Eventually, Professor Calnan mentioned the term 'AVM' – arteriovenous malformation – which I'd never heard before. AVMs happen when a group of blood vessels in your body forms incorrectly. Normally, arteries carrying blood under pressure divide down, reduce in size and pressure, and form capillaries; blood then returns via the capillaries to the veins. In a high-flow AVM like mine, the mass of blood vessels that form run from artery straight to vein (doctors call this an arteriovenous shunt), missing capillaries out completely. The veins, wide and elastic, fill with blood, still under pressure. This can increase until the vein ruptures and bleeding occurs under arterial pressure. If there is a lot of flow through an AVM, the heart may strain to keep up, leading to heart failure.

No one knows why AVMs form, but they are best thought of as birthmarks that can occur anywhere in the body. They're thought to affect approximately 1.4 in every 100,000 people. The biggest concern is that AVMs will cause uncontrolled bleeding – or haemorrhage. Fewer than four per cent of AVMs haemorrhage, but those that do can have a severe, even fatal, effect. Death as a direct result of an AVM happens in about one per cent of people with AVMs.

Initially, there had been no obvious sign of an AVM, Professor Calnan told us, but on subsequent testing that had now changed. I had no idea what any of it meant nor how serious it could be, and it wasn't until later I discovered it was a rare vascular anomaly that was notoriously difficult to manage.

He wanted to do another angiogram to establish the size of the AVM and to understand what vessels were feeding it. I was in hospital overnight, had a groin puncture and was injected full of dye for the angiogram. Afterwards, Professor Calnan told me I was going to need an operation to remove the AVM and that he needed an excellent vascular surgeon to do it. The vascular surgeon would be required to ligate or tie off major blood vessels in the head and neck, which involved the greatest risk. That's when he introduced us to John Lynn.

Professor Calnan also said that a few weeks before the operation I would need to have a procedure called an embolisation, which would block the blood vessels supplying the abnormal growth and reduce the size of the AVM pre-op. This technique was fairly new at the time, and Professor David Allison, who would perform the operation on me, was a pioneer of the procedure.

In October 1980, I went to the Hammersmith for the first of several embolisation procedures I would have over the next few years. Embolisation is similar to an angiogram. Under x-ray guidance, it involves a catheter being inserted into an artery in the groin and manipulated into the blood vessels supplying the AVM. Spring coils and other foreign material, including absorbable gelatine sponge, hypertonic dextrose and polyvinyl alcohol, are then pushed or injected through the catheter to block these blood vessels off in order to reduce the excessive blood flow.

This all took place while I was still awake – no anaesthetic other than a local in the groin. I lay there, staring up at the scanning machine above me that showed what was going on inside, and watched the coils ascending through the arteries up to my head.

Professor Allison injected some dye and I watched it on the screen, flaring up like a supernova – all these tiny stars just glowing. I watched as he got the coils ready and squashed them into a particular area in my head. It was important to get it exactly right because if it blocked the wrong artery, it could deprive the blood supply to the eye and I'd end up irreversibly blind. There was also the small matter of blood supply to the brain if he got it wrong … that's why I had to be awake. Now and then, Professor Allison would lean over and say, 'Can you still see?' to reassure himself he'd got the right spot.

I was in a heightened state of tension because, at any second, that could be it. When he said the word 'freeze', I had to pick a spot on the ceiling and stare at it and not even blink. Then he'd say 'relax', and I'd relax and he'd inject some more dye and spring coils. Whenever he injected the dye, I could feel my entire face warming up. The actual coils themselves felt like sticking your head in a beehive and getting stung over and over.

~

Case report: He first noticed a pulsatile swelling affecting the left side of the face at the age of 14 when he was admitted to another hospital and underwent surgery...

Case notes (1981): Ligation of left lingual artery. Ligation of right facial artery. Excision of fistula. Vessels penetrating left mandible. Lesion excised, query left nerve damage both facial and left lingual artery divided and ligated. Blood loss approx. 1200 millilitres.

~

Three months later, in February 1981, I had major head and neck surgery in an attempt to remove the AVM. The doctors made an incision from ear to ear, flipped back the skin (like taking off a face mask), scraped the mandible and tied off the main feeder vessels into the AVM, the idea being that restricting the blood flow to the area would deprive the cells of oxygen and therefore the mass of abnormal tissues would shrink because the cells would die.

The vascular surgeon John Lynn told me later it was a bloodbath in the operating theatre. He said the body has this survival mechanism where it realises it's not getting blood to an area, so it opens up other dormant or collateral vessels that start feeding blood to the area that's deprived. So, as he had begun ligating the blood vessels to stop the blood supply getting to the area, other collateral vessels had opened up. He ended up chasing these vessels around my head as blood pumped out all over the place.

The complexities of the operation also meant a higher chance of mishaps, like when the surgeon accidentally cut the mandibular branch of the facial nerve. I was left paralysed on the left side of the face and lip. It felt (and still feels) like I'd had a dental injection prior to having a filling, only it's permanent.

John Lynn also told us that if they had to do another operation, I would probably bleed to death, since those collateral vessels kept opening up. Still, being a teenager, I didn't take it that seriously. I couldn't contemplate it happening again – nor that I might die if it did.

Within a few weeks of the operation, I returned to Glasgow because I was sitting my higher school examinations in a few months. By this time, Mum and George had moved to Oxfordshire as George had joined the Royal Air Force (RAF). George wanted a better life for us and to get away from Drumchapel, so he left his job as a delivery driver for a bakery company and joined the RAF as a military policeman. His first posting was RAF Benson in Oxfordshire, which is only about an hour and a half from London. Ultimately, it meant I was closer to Hammersmith Hospital for follow-up appointments.

But, in the meantime, it was back to Glasgow to stay with Granny in Possilpark for those final three or four months of the school year. Charlie wasn't there – I'm not sure why. One of his stints in jail, most likely, and that was certainly a relief. I was pumped full of drugs after the operation – strong painkillers and yellow tablets to help me sleep. My head felt as if it was going to burst. Night time was the worst. It was as if I had a heart in my head, beating and throbbing, causing great pain. Somehow, I managed to attend school every day, even though I had to catch two different buses across the city to get there.

Looking back, I can't believe I managed it with the pain, the strong drugs and a new scar from ear to ear. I don't know how I survived. But I sat my higher school examinations in May 1981 and soon after joined my parents in Oxfordshire.

CHAPTER 4

A Downward Spiral at Boarding School

Our new house, on the base at RAF Benson in Oxfordshire, was a far cry from the close we had shared with six other families in Drumchapel. This was a fancy detached three-bedroom house with a back and front garden. The base was home to the Queen's flight aircraft – both fixed-wing planes and helicopters belonging to the royal family, prime minister and ministers of the UK government.

George told us that one of his duties as a military policeman was to be part of an advance party, whereby he would go to places a few days ahead of the Queen arriving. He and another colleague had a critical duty – to assess if a toilet was suitable for the Queen to use, should she need one. George would go into the proposed toilet. His colleague would close the toilet door and stand outside (pretending to be the Queen's bodyguard). George would use one of those plastic washing-up squeeze-type bottles (full of water). He would then squirt the contents of the water into the toilet bowl. The toilet would only pass the test for the Queen's usage if his colleague could not hear the sound of water hitting the toilet bowl. If the policeman outside the door *could* hear the sound of water squirting into the toilet bowl, that toilet could never be used for the Queen – because no one could ever hear the Queen pee.

How true that story was I do not know, but George loved to tell it – regaling people with it was his favourite party piece.

Not long after I arrived at the house on the base at RAF Benson, my higher school examination results arrived in the mail. Despite the fact I'd returned to Scotland after the operation and put in the best effort I could under the circumstances, I only scraped through, which was not good enough to get into university. But since my plan had always been to go to university, I wanted to go on and do my A-levels. I'd always had a curious mind and was interested in the way things worked. In the Drum, from around the age of twelve, I would go to the library, searching for Einstein's papers on the general theory of relativity and any books I could find about time and space, how the universe worked – how anything worked really. It was always science-based material I was interested in, so I knew that would be the direction I'd go in at university, but I had to get the A-levels first.

We started exploring local schools in Oxfordshire, but, within a few weeks, we heard that George's next posting was going to be in Germany at RAF Brüggen (home to fighter aircraft of the RAF). So, we had a discussion around what to do about my schooling. Should I go to Germany with my family and find a school there, or have a look at UK boarding school options, which the air force would pay for? We decided on the latter so I could focus on my studies and not have to move again. It was quite incredible. Only a few months earlier, I was at a council-run school in the Drum and now we were considering a posh boarding school, culturally light-years away from my upbringing on a council estate in Glasgow.

We settled on Brockenhurst College in Hampshire and I started there in September 1981. Southampton, famous for its port and maritime heritage, was the nearest big city. The small boarding house I stayed at was called Culverley House. Many of the other students there were the children of non-commissioned officers like George, or commissioned officers, and their parents were stationed all over the world. Some of them had been there since the start of secondary school at age twelve, as their parents would move around every two or three years. They either went to the nearby secondary college or the older students, like me, to Brockenhurst College for A-levels. It was a couple of kilometres from the boarding house and we would walk to school every day.

I was in the sixth form and I seemed to fit quite easily into boarding school life. Maybe the skills gained while surviving the hard streets of the Drum enabled me to slot into this comfortable environment. I had this broad Glaswegian accent, which very few people understood. I could tell because they would emit this nervous laugh every time I spoke. And with a scar from ear to ear, people probably thought I was a gangster.

The work ethic I had developed doing my paper round in Drumchapel followed me here. To earn some cash, I picked up litter in the college grounds for 2.50 pounds an hour every Saturday morning. Although in time, I found a more creative way to generate money – perhaps exacerbating my gangster image – by building a small brewery in the attic of the boarding house, along with my best friend, Tony Adolph, and selling homebrew to the students. Our side gig was selling the leftover sediment, which was highly concentrated and therefore extremely alcoholic. It was very popular among the student body, as was our other business: selling pornographic magazines, including a 'buy two, get one free' special offer.

The teachers had no clue what we were up to and they never did find out. We'd climb up into the attic, which was quite warm and comfortable, and run our clandestine business. This went on for months, right up until exam time when it seemed prudent to stop.

In addition to our business enterprises, Tony Adolph and I had a lot of fun together. Culverley House was in the New Forest, so we would take all the other kids out and go for mad runs through the marshy fields and woodlands, spotting ponies and maybe even a donkey. I also got into some orienteering too – the New Forest setting was perfect for such activities.

Alongside these healthier pursuits, there was a lot of drinking, to which the teachers just seemed to turn a blind eye. Although I didn't drink alcohol daily, I was one for massive weekend binges when it was quiet around the boarding house. No one had ever advised me that I shouldn't drink alcohol. In hindsight, given my diagnosis and increased risk of bleeds, who knows what damage I might have been doing.

Most of the students went to stay with relatives or friends on the weekend. Often there were only two or three of us left. Sometimes for the shorter holidays or long weekends, I'd stay with my aunt Rose-Ann and uncle Keith, who were also in the army, based in Andover, not far from the boarding school. For Christmas and summer holidays, I'd go to Germany. But otherwise, most weekends I would be at the boarding house looking for distractions.

A teacher at the boarding house was a member of the Young Farmers Club, an organisation for young people who were interested in agriculture. One day, they had a party in a big barn. Tony Adolph and I, along with a few other sixth formers, went along with the teacher. It was an all-afternoon, into-the-evening type of affair. By mid-evening I'd had twenty pints of lager and a number of shots, and I was still dancing. Eventually, though, almost comatose, I collapsed in a heap on the dance floor. My body couldn't handle the sheer amount of alcohol I had consumed, and I was vomiting up blood by that point. The teacher called an ambulance, and I was rushed to Southampton General Hospital where I had my stomach pumped.

Although I had physically healed from my operation and was no longer taking sleeping pills or painkillers, I had never taken the time to heal mentally. I had never really addressed the post-traumatic stress from my early life with Big Jerry, either. Consuming vast amounts of alcohol was my way of coping with life and it seemed to numb the mental pain I was clearly in. I had all sorts of emotions and a great deal of confusion. I didn't really know who I was nor what I was up to. Alcohol was a crutch and I had no control over it.

The other thing weighing on my mind was the fact that the swelling on my face from after the operation had not gone away. In fact, it was getting bigger. As I grew older and my body developed with all the hormones of puberty, the swelling continued to worsen to the point that it began to squash my left eye. I think that's when I developed the ability to put things in boxes and lock them away, just to cope. After being told I might die if I ever needed another operation, feelings of immense fear developed within my psyche. But at the tender age of nineteen, I just packed them away and continued on with life … and drinking.

It wasn't just fear of what might happen to me physically. It was a totally debilitating fear of what the future might hold and a sense of desperation. Every day was mentally exhausting. I had little hope for the future – how could I think about a career or a serious girlfriend or getting married one day when I was walking around feeling like the Elephant Man, with this ever-expanding growth on my face? No one would ever love me or give me a job… What was I doing in life? Where was I going? What was the point of it all if life was going to continue like this? This kind of circular thinking was getting worse and worse. I didn't know how to stop the spiralling thoughts, other than to get as drunk as possible.

I was becoming consumed with my own negativity, and I couldn't discuss it with anyone. There seemed to be no way of stopping it. I also knew I'd done really badly in the recent exams and that thought was adding to my distress – failure yet again… Then one day, I just decided to end it. I couldn't take it anymore and there seemed no point in continuing. I polished off a fair amount of alcohol and swallowed a bottle of painkillers the doctors had given me after the operation. It was the weekend and there weren't many other students around.

Some hours later, another student found me lying on my bed. He asked me what was going on, and I managed to tell him, though I must have been mumbling and sounding confused. He rushed off to get one of the teachers, who called an ambulance and then took me to the toilet and told me to try and make myself throw up, which I managed to do.

I ended up at Southampton General Hospital again. As I lay there in my hospital bed, with a big tube in my stomach and drips all around me, two nurses were having a conversation as they carried out the stomach pump procedure. It was about their forthcoming holiday in Ibiza and how they were looking forward to it so much. As I was being sick every few minutes, I thought to myself, '*Hey, life really does go on whether I am alive or dead – no one really cares.*'

It is difficult to explain to anyone why you would want to kill yourself. As a living entity, your instinct is always to survive.

However, in your darkest days, you end up in a sort of inward spiral and consumed by your own negativity that you cannot get out of or stop. Your headspace is consumed with such circular thoughts that you think the only option is death.

But I didn't die. I survived and moved on … locking it away like everything else and getting on with things because that's what you do. Exams were over, so I ended up moving to Germany when I was discharged from hospital. The doctors had wanted to refer me to a local psychiatrist. I told them I would see a psychiatrist in Germany through the air force, which I did, but I was given no real diagnosis or treatment plan. I'm sure the psychiatrist just said there was nothing really wrong with me. That was in the good old days when they'd just as soon prescribe a stiff whisky than anything more useful or appropriate.

As I got off the plane in Germany, Mum simply said, 'I love you and I'm just pleased you're home. It doesn't matter what's happened or what you've done – it's just good to have you home.' God bless her.

CHAPTER 5

Avoiding the Stiff Inn in Germany

Royal Air Force Brüggen, where George was stationed, was a massive camp on the Dutch-German border that first became active in the 1950s as NATO forces expanded in Europe. It had nuclear weapons and fighter aircraft such as Jaguars and Tornados.

It was June 1983 when I arrived in Germany. My parents were living in a little modern terrace house about fifteen kilometres away from the base in Donderberg in the Netherlands. It was a satellite town just across the German border, where they stationed married couples and families. Unfortunately, that meant every time you wanted to get to the camp, you had to go through the border checkpoints.

My exam results from boarding school arrived soon after I did and, not surprisingly, they were so low that they were not good enough to get into any university. The curriculum I had studied in Scotland was very different to England, which took a while to get used to. But that wasn't the real issue. It was my mental state that was the problem – specifically, not knowing what I was doing nor what the future held.

Being in Germany with my family did seem to help though. I felt more grounded, and, over the next couple of months, I took some time to decide what I was going to do. I was still keen on going to university so I decided to attend a local English school and re-sit the A-level exams.

~

Case notes: In 1984 aged 19 years he was admitted to hospital following a brisk haemorrhage from between the lower left incisor and premolar teeth but did not require transfusion or surgical intervention.

One evening, not long after I'd started back at school, I felt a trickle of blood in my mouth and immediately my body went into survival mode. The doctors had warned me about potential bleeds because of the situation with my arteries and veins and the AVM causing them to become thin and weak. When they had first told me I did not really appreciate the danger or magnitude of the condition, although my mum realised the enormity of what was going on. Rather than walking around like a ticking time bomb, I was more of a throbbing time bomb that could explode at any time. She was obviously worried and played it down so she wouldn't alarm me.

But by that stage I knew it could be fatal, so I grabbed a hand towel and put it in my mouth and clamped my hand over it to hold it firmly in place. Mum and George were in the living room watching TV after dinner. As soon as I entered the room, they could see how bad the situation was and how distressed I was with blood pumping out of my face.

It was dark outside as we rushed to the car, Mum carrying Paul, who was a toddler at the time. Sharon, who would've been twelve, must have been at a friend's for dinner or an extracurricular activity as she wasn't there, but she remembers the shock of arriving back home after we'd left and finding blood all over the bathroom. It must have left her distraught, facing that alone and not knowing what the outcome for her brother might be.

Mum and George knew they had to get me straight to RAF Brüggen rather than the local Dutch hospital which would not know my background (and we did not speak any Dutch anyway). When I had first arrived, Mum had taken me to the camp to see the dentist and the doctor – just in case anything like this happened – so the doctors there knew my medical history.

We sped towards the border, knowing we would have to go through two checkpoints: the Dutch border first, then across a little no-man's-land, like a dual carriageway, to the German border. When we arrived at the first checkpoint, George and Mum tried to explain to the Dutch border police (without speaking Dutch) that it was a medical emergency. But the policeman still said, 'Can I have your passports, please?' George, who was really not fond of the sight of blood, was rushing around trying to get the passports out of the glove compartment. Mum was screaming and shouting, 'My son is going to bleed to death. We need to get on!' Eventually, the guards looked into the back seat of the car to see me lying in a pool of my own blood and immediately sent us on our way.

At RAF Brüggen, they called the maxillofacial surgeons at RAF Wegberg – the RAF military hospital – to say we were on our way. Fortunately, the bleeding stopped fairly quickly after we arrived and I didn't need treatment other than to be monitored, though they kept me there for a few days after everything settled down, just in case.

When I had recovered, one of the medics, a Scottish guy, took great delight in pointing out this little bar to me. It was in a hut outside the medical centre. He told me if somebody died in the camp, they put the body in a frozen container in the little hut, which they called the Stiff Inn. He said, 'Jerry, you're very fortunate because you'd have been put in there had you died. That's where the bodies go … and there's a bar there as well. You could have ended up in the Stiff Inn, with everyone having a drink for you.' That's some black humour for you – trust the Scots!

After this bleeding episode, the RAF moved us from Donderberg to a house at RAF Brüggen in case another such episode happened, so we could get to the medical centre quickly.

~

That was the first of several bleeds over the next few years that would increase in intensity and, in time, come to threaten my life. Meanwhile, the swelling on the left side of my face was getting bigger all the time and becoming a purple-blue colour – probably the result of the AVM becoming even more vascular in nature.

Despite that, I enjoyed my time in Germany. I made some good friends through the school and at the Brüggen Youth Club. That's where I met Mark, who became a very good friend. Many years later, I was his best man. Mark and I had some good times together, many of which involved drinking, which was a strong part of the culture on the base.

One memory of our drinking remains in technicolour glory in my mind. The morning after a long, alcohol-fuelled party, I was sitting on the front steps at the hospital, RAF Wegberg. A hangover was just setting in. Mark had popped into the hospital to get a can of Coke from the vending machine. After a night of drinking, we liked to drink flat Coke (flat because it would not bloat your stomach) and top up our sugar levels further with a Mars Bar. As I waited for Mark to come back, who should come up the steps but the maxillofacial surgeon, who was a group captain in the RAF. He was over six feet tall and towered over me. I must have been speaking utter drivel at him because of the state I was in. He truly thought I was having another bleed and that's why I was at the hospital.

Other nights when we were drinking at Brüggen, rather than go home, Mark and I would sneak into the male accommodation block for the RAF personnel who slept in large dormitories. More often than not there was a bed not being used, as personnel were out on RAF exercises or home in the UK visiting family and friends. We would then sneak out before sunrise, thinking we were so clever – aha, got away with it again!

After another drunken adventure at Brüggen, Mark and I were catching the night bus back to Donderberg and we were legless. Just for kicks, we dropped our pants and flashed our buttocks out the back window of the bus to the cars behind as we went through the German-Dutch border. Imagine my absolute shock and horror when I got home to find it was Mum and George in the car behind. Mum said she knew it was me because she'd recognise those buttocks anywhere.

~

I was working towards my A-levels but, again, the syllabus was completely different to that of both Scotland and the school in Hampshire. When my results came in, I still didn't score high enough to get into the university courses I wanted to do, so I re-sat the exams for a third time a few months later. Finally, in March 1985, I managed to get sufficient grades in mathematics, physics and chemistry – the subjects I needed for university.

I still hadn't settled on what I would study. I was thinking about becoming an engineer or a pilot and joining the air force. I was also thinking about doing medicine because I had spent so much time in hospitals. I was interested in astrophysics and astronomy, and in nuclear fusion and how nuclear fusion reactions power the sun.

In the end I was offered a position in several degree courses – anatomy at Bristol University (a precursor for medicine), electrical engineering at Newcastle University and nuclear engineering at Manchester University. I decided to go for the latter since I had always had a fascination with all things nuclear.

The new term would not start until October 1985, so I had a few months to kill. I was keen to earn some cash rather than sponge money from my parents. I saw an advertisement for a toilet cleaner with a squadron that serviced Tornado and Jaguar aircraft. In addition, the job involved cleaning up aircraft oil leaks in the hangars. This involved covering the oil spillages with chicken excrement and leaving it until the oil had been absorbed – then disposing of the saturated chicken shit. As I waited for the chicken shit to be absorbed, I used the time to clean the toilets. Rather than call myself a toilet cleaner, I called myself a sanitary hygienist. After a while I received a promotion to look after additional toilets so I promoted myself to *chief* sanitary hygienist.

On my last day on the job, I decided I would play a joke on the aircrew of the squadron. Being the smartass I was, I put cling film on the toilet seats, then put the cover down so you couldn't see it.

When the aircrew came rushing in to use the toilets after many hours in the air flying their fighter jets, they sat down to enjoy a bowel movement and, well, let's just say they ended up in the shit.

My days as chief sanitary hygienist at RAF Brüggen were over. I was moving on to bigger and better things … but, as I was about to discover, it would be far from smooth sailing.

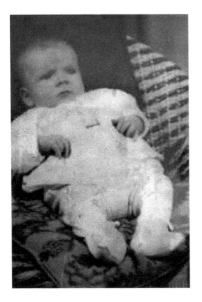

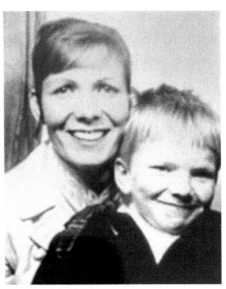

Serious baby, born
into chaos.

Happy times with my mum.

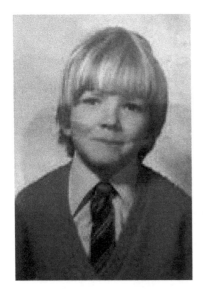

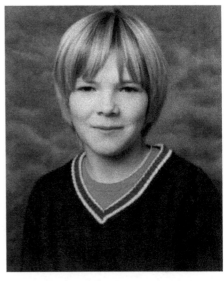

St Pius Primary. Smiling
like an angel, hiding
the pain within.

St Pius Secondary. Turning past
struggles into chess victories.

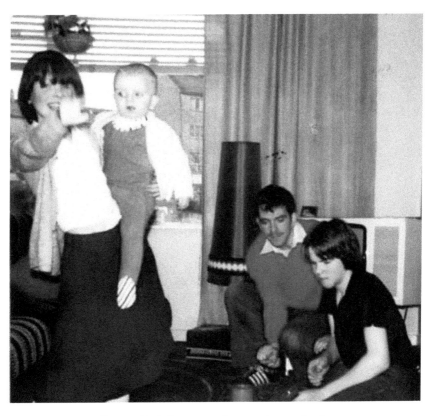

Sharon, Paul, George and me – a happy family.

PART 2

FINDING THE WILL TO SURVIVE

CHAPTER 6

Misadventures at University

The bus left Germany on a Friday morning headed for Belgium, then on to Zeebrugge for the ferry trip across the English Channel. I arrived in Manchester on Saturday morning, twenty-four hours after I'd hugged my family goodbye. I had two suitcases to last me for the duration of my three-year degree: one filled with clothes, the other with pots, pans and cutlery.

Feeling a little lost and wondering where the hell I was supposed to be, I eventually found my way to the halls of residence where I was to live for the next couple of years. The halls consisted of a series of little apartments in blocks of eight with a shared toilet, bathroom and kitchen/living room area.

My parents didn't have much money in those days, so I didn't have to pay a penny for my university education or accommodation – it was all free courtesy of the government. One of the first things to take care of was setting up a bank account at the nearby NatWest (National Westminster Bank) branch so I could receive my living allowance in the form of government cheques. I could never have gone to university if we'd had to pay, and I'm very grateful for that opportunity.

University life suited me. It was fun hanging out with the other students in Oak House, the block I lived in with seven other people, and I enjoyed my course, which, happily, led to me passing all my first-year exams. I didn't have any health dramas that first year either, so it was a good year all round. Unfortunately, that was not to be the case in my second year…

One day, early in that second year, when I was heading from the campus back to my accommodation, I noticed a metallic taste in my mouth. It was blood, and it was rapidly spraying out of my mouth and all over my face, neck and clothes. I was at the traffic lights, waiting for the 'walk' light to go green. By the time I had walked across the road, I was so saturated in blood that people passing by thought I'd been in a hit-and-run accident. Someone told me to lie down on the pavement in the recovery position while a friend from the halls of residence called an ambulance.

It was distressing not being able to explain to anyone what was going on. I couldn't take my hand away from my mouth or the blood would spray out. Holding my hand there stemmed the flow somewhat. It seemed like forever, but eventually I heard the ambulance siren and a sense of relief washed over me.

When the ambulance arrived at Manchester Royal Infirmary, the doctors in the emergency department didn't really know what to do with me. By then the bleeding had stopped and I was able to tell them to contact the Hammersmith to speak to the vascular surgeon there, John Lynn, who could explain what was going on. But since the bleeding had stopped, they just took my details and told me I could go home!

'*It's just as well I had some cash to get back to the halls of residence*,' I thought to myself as I sat in the back of a taxi. Imagine the stares I would have encountered if I had to catch the bus with my clothes covered in congealed blood. When I got home, I phoned John Lynn myself to tell him what had happened, and he insisted I immediately get myself to the Casualty Department of the Hammersmith Hospital.

With no dilly-dallying, I threw some clothes and personal items in a bag and jumped on a bus to the train station. A small clot had formed where the bleeding had originated from in my mouth, and I was acutely aware of it all the way to London. I knew that if I touched it with my tongue, or had anything to eat or drink, it could burst and another bleeding session would transpire. I was petrified, thinking, '*Shit ... I hope this doesn't blow!*' It was a good three hours by train from Manchester to London. I knew that if I had another bleed on the journey, there wouldn't be time for a blood transfusion and I would bleed to death.

When I arrived at the Hammersmith, John Lynn organised another embolisation to get on top of it. After the procedure, I wasn't allowed out of bed for a day or so because blood clots might form after the groin puncture, so I had to stay there for at least a couple of days. Then more tests were required to see if everything had settled down.

Throughout those first few days, they plied me with heavy painkillers to help with the bee-sting-like pain from having the coils inserted. I was in the hospital for a week, and then I had a week of recovery at my aunt Rose-Ann and uncle Keith's place in Andover. I just chilled out in the garden and watched TV, resting and getting myself organised. I couldn't really eat much at the time – nothing hard because that could trigger another bleed. I'd eat baby food like Farley's Rusks, which were hard and crumbly, and full of vitamins and proteins. I would dunk them in tea or hot milk to make them softer. And then it was back to university, hoping for the best.

~

> **Case notes (1989):** Bleeding slowly for the past hour (5 am). Sudden drop in blood pressure, cold and sweating. Transfused 2 units. (10.30 am) bleeding now ceased. Discussed with Prof Allison all feeder vessels have been embolised. Further angio would be unhelpful. Discussed with Mr Lynn and agreed that further embolisation would not help – unresectable.

That wasn't the only bleed or embolisation I had during those years, but they blur together in my mind. By the end of my third year at university, I'd had as many embolisations as they could give me. There are only so many steel coils that can be inserted into someone's head and neck, after all.

I remember another time I was at the Hammersmith, though, because there was a young Irish nurse looking after me during the night. I remember her voice and that Irish lilt, which had a calming effect on me. She sat with me all night even though her shift had finished. Another massive bleed had occurred. After several hours it had stopped, but when I took the bandage away, it took the sealed top off and the bleeding started up yet again. It was as if the Irish nurse, who was much the same age as me, thought I was going to bleed to death and didn't want me to be alone when it happened. I could actually *feel* her realisation that I might die … because they couldn't do any more embolisations to help the situation. I either stopped bleeding or I bled to death.

I remember looking out the window. It was dark outside, but

there was an orange glow from the street lights and I just stared at that light, kind of transfixed. I was absolutely exhausted, with nothing more to give after bleeding for several hours straight. When it started again, I almost gave up. I remember thinking, *'Fuck this, I just can't go on like this again.'* But it helped having her there – this calming presence. She sat there all night and didn't leave me. I must have fallen asleep at some point, and the next morning she was gone.

~

In my final year at university, I ventured out of the halls of residence to live in a share house in Withington, South Manchester. It was a shithole with green and white mould up the walls and across the ceiling. There were so many students living there along with the guy who owned it. It was a horrible environment to live in, but, in those days, you took what you could get.

One of the guys who lived there was Tony T., who was doing a PhD in history, and we became good friends. One night after we'd been out drinking, we had this bright idea. It was based around the fact that I'd never had a serious girlfriend and wondered if I ever would. I'd never had sex with anyone, and, as a young man, it plays tricks on your mind. I wondered what options were available to me when my face was so badly swollen. Who would have sex with me? There was clearly not going to be an immediate physical attraction on the girl's part. I could die at any time from a bleed and still not have experienced sex.

Tony T. had been telling me about his experiences with his girlfriend, and, in particular, about 'fanny farts'. I thought to myself, *'Fanny farts – what the hell is that all about?'* Having never had sex, I had no idea there was such a thing. In my naive mind, I was seriously questioning what biological evolutionary advantage fanny farts would have. Of course, from a physics point of view – and I was a science man after all – I guessed a piston going up and down in a cylinder built up pressure with trapped air needing to escape, perhaps with a large explosion. Could fanny farts be some sort of weapon of mass destruction? Good grief – the next thing Tony would be telling me was that a vagina spoke to him.

By the time we had this bizarre conversation, rather a lot of alcohol had been consumed. And that's when Tony suggested I should have sex with a prostitute – which seemed like a good idea at the time. So, like the bright sparks we were, we headed out, drunk off our heads, to the redlight district, which is down by the canals in Manchester, among the warehouses and cobbled laneways that were once at the heart of a thriving cotton industry in the region.

When we arrived down by the canals, sure enough, two ladies of the night appeared from the dark alleyways and called out to Tony and me to negotiate a price. One of them took me by the hand and led me down a dark, cobbled laneway. But just as I got around the corner with her and my pants were down around my ankles, I heard this voice shout out, 'Stop, stop, stop!' Tony T. appeared, running down the alleyway. His conscience had clearly got the better of him and he couldn't allow it to happen. Next thing he started shouting, 'Oh, he's not well, he's got this medical condition...' in a bid to explain why we were backing out of the deal. So that was the end of that ... I hoicked up my trousers and Tony and I staggered home. The next day I woke up with a hangover, thinking, '*What the fuck just happened there?*'

The truth is, what happened there was quite understandable. Knowing you might not live for very long doesn't exactly lead to stable mental health and the best of choices, especially when you're a young guy at university with a disfigured face who has never had sex and might never get the chance to do so.

Quite a few years later, I did experience fanny farts in action for myself. And it is indeed a phenomenon.

∼

That same year at university, since I was fascinated by all things astronomy, space and time dimensions, as a bit of fun I tried to use applied mathematics to prove a theorem for time travel. I had it all planned out in this red folder (which I still have today). I even considered doing it for my third-year project, but, unfortunately, it wasn't practical. In the end, the actual project I handed in was for a type of demand valve for oxygen delivery. I made a working prototype and I went to the Manchester Royal Infirmary to research it. It was like a demand valve that divers use in oxygen tanks and that they use in blood transfusions for babies. I used it in a mobile oxygen unit for elderly people so that they could move around. So, despite some of my crazy behaviour and questionable choices at that time, like my misadventure with the prostitute, I was also doing some good work.

I ended up getting a first for that project. In 1988, I left Manchester University with an upper second-class honours degree in nuclear engineering. It was time to start my career ... but who knew what the future might hold for someone like me?

CHAPTER 7

Rugby, Partying and a Police Escort

After graduation in 1988, I was accepted into the graduate training program with General Electric Company (GEC). It was a two-year graduate apprenticeship based in Rugby, Warwickshire, a market town near Birmingham in the centre of England renowned for being the birthplace of the game of rugby.

I stayed in a hotel for the first few weeks after I arrived, then I moved into a room in a shared house on Sun Street. A guy who worked at GEC, Bill Armstrong, owned the house and rented out two rooms to me and another graduate trainee. Bill was the manufacturing manager, only a few years older than me, but already in a senior position running the business unit.

There were graduates from all over the country in the training program. We were to spend the next two years shuffling through all the different departments, learning about construction, manufacturing and engineering, and specifically, what was involved in building power stations, steam turbines, generators and so on.

When I arrived, I still had my two big suitcases, one with all my cooking utensils. Not that I used them much; I was always eating out of a pot in those days. My thinking was: Why create more dirty dishes when you didn't need to? I really wasn't into cooking, so I spent half my life at the local kebab shop. I'd drive past the shop, wave at the shop owner, and, by the time I'd parked the car, he'd have a big doner kebab and chips ready to go.

At one point, they sent us to East Warwickshire College for six months, to learn how to do sheet metal work and manufacturing. I'm not a very practical person, so I struggled with this course. I didn't even know how to use the tools they provided in the toolbox. The guy who was running the course thought I was dyslexic, or whatever the equivalent is in terms of hands-on tradie-type skills, but I'm just not practical. I'm quite happy to break something up, but I can't put it back together again.

I did gradually get into some fitness there though, which helped counter all the kebabs and booze I was imbibing. Throughout those six months, I became friends with the college's physical education trainer, Steve Rigg. He eventually went on to become the best man at my wedding…

Socially, I was thriving at GEC. By the end of the first year, I was elected as chairperson for the Student and Graduate Training Association (SAGTA) and in charge of all social events. We organised a big twenty-four-hour dartathon at the local pub, among other things.

I also made some other good friends in addition to Steve Rigg. There was a fellow Scotsman, Tom Richardson, and another guy, Richard Drabble, who both started at GEC the same day as me. Richard was one of the Gruesome Foursome, which also comprised me and two young women we met through Steve Rigg – Adrienne and Sarah. They were both doing a marketing and business management course at Rugby College and we had a great time hanging out together. I had this yellow Mitsubishi

Colt, which was falling apart, and we called it the Mobile Coffin because it was essentially a death trap. The windows didn't work – you'd wind them down and they'd come down at an angle. But we didn't care. We'd load up the Mobile Coffin and head out on day trips, for picnics and to parties.

I was in my element. Life was cruising along just fine in terms of my working life at GEC and the social environment in Rugby … that is, until the next medical episode that threatened my life.

~

Case notes: Angiography carried out in February 1990 showed an extensive vascular malformation, centred predominantly around and within the body of the left mandible which was fed by numerous ectatic arteries including the right lingual, right maxillary, right transverse facial and also the left ophthalmic artery (supplying the lesion via nasociliary anastomoses).

Most Thursdays in Rugby involved a large turnout at the local pubs. But on Thursday, 22 February 1990, my thoughts were of the weekend ahead, since I had a big one planned. On Friday I was looking forward to seeing the David Lynch movie *Blue Velvet* at the Warwick Arts Centre, then some of us were heading to London on Saturday. On Sunday afternoon, there was a leaving party for a guy named Steve Cook, who was off to New York to work. If I made it back to Rugby by nine o'clock on Sunday evening, the plan was to go swimming to 'sweat out' the hard stuff before Monday back at work.

On Thursday, Steve Rigg and I met up at a local pub, the William Webb Ellis, with the usual faces. As part of our health and fitness program, Perrier water was our tipple of choice that evening, since we were both turning into fat gits thanks to years of alcoholic abuse. However, we did indulge in a cognac or two back at Steve's house after the pub.

It was around half past one in the morning when I arrived home, ready to crash out. I quietly entered the house so as not to awaken Bill Armstrong. As I brushed my teeth, I felt a trickle of blood oozing out from the side of my mouth. '*Oh, hell no, here we go again,*' I thought with alarm. Its pace quickened and blood soon began to pump out under arterial pressure, flowing out like a heavy nosebleed. There was no time to give in to the panic I was feeling – I needed to keep myself alive. I grabbed a towel and clamped it into my mouth with my right hand. Ripping a page from my diary, which contained some information about my condition as well as the names and phone numbers of medical staff in London, I headed out to the car, knowing I needed to get to hospital as quickly as possible. There was no time to awaken Bill – he would wake up in the morning to see the bloodbath in his bathroom.

I thrashed my car all the way to the Hospital of St Cross, with full-beam headlights on, steering with my left hand while my right hand stayed in my mouth. (Fortunately, I am left-handed.) No doubt I well exceeded the legal speed limit on that journey. The car brakes screeched as I skidded to a halt outside the casualty entrance. It was silent, dimly lit and with no sign of life, which concerned me. Thankfully, a nurse soon appeared and asked me what had happened. Unfortunately, with my hand in my mouth and large clots of blood flowing out, I couldn't speak, so I handed her the page from my diary.

She gave me some absorbent pads and lay me on a bed until a young doctor appeared. Soon the bleeding eased and slowly stopped. At one point, another of the nurses looking after me asked if I recognised her, but I did not. She explained she was the wife of one of my fellow GEC graduate trainees and we'd met at a Christmas dinner.

The doctor was keen to get a photograph of me, as an arteriovenous malformation was rare indeed, he said. '*You're telling me!*' I thought to myself. '*Just get me to the Hammersmith,*' I pleaded silently. I obliged them anyway, my face and clothes covered in blood as the nurse took a snapshot, but the camera didn't work. As they discussed the technical hitch, I was left to my own devices, again desperately thinking, '*Will you just call the Hammersmith now, please?!*'

The casualty doctor eventually gave up on his hopes of getting a good shot of my face and telephoned the Hammersmith. He informed the duty doctor there about the situation, and I couldn't believe the response. The duty doctor told him there were no beds available at the Hammersmith, and, also, my records showed that after all the embolisations I'd already had, the medical problem could not be solved. He suggested I therefore stay overnight at St Cross to see what happened.

I shook my head in disbelief and suggested the casualty doctor call John Lynn directly instead. He did, only to find John was on holiday. By this time, I was getting seriously concerned. I knew that if the bleeding started again, I could bleed to death. I stressed this point to the casualty doctor yet again, and he agreed to try the

Hammersmith one more time. Finally, after much discussion and time wasted, it was agreed that I would travel to the Hammersmith that night.

To add to all this, there happened to be a national ambulance strike going on. How would I get to the Hammersmith Hospital, which was a good hour and a half away in London? After some investigating, the medical staff informed me that an army Land Rover ambulance would transport me to London led by a police escort. When they arrived, the doctor suggested to the police that I should lie horizontally in the back of their Jaguar, since the small clot that had formed in my mouth could easily be dislodged through the movement of my head or body in a bumpy Land Rover, which would restart the bleeding. Unfortunately, this was not approved because of police insurance policies, and I was gently transferred to the ambulance with a young army medic accompanying me plus the driver.

I still had the gauze in my mouth, half inside and half outside. The blood had congealed, and I lay motionless, terrified any movement would initiate a bleed. I kept my eyes strictly fixed on the light bulb of the white roof, noticing that the smell of army greens was only surpassed by the horrible smell of congealed blood in and outside my mouth.

The journey was slow and bumpy, but the medic reassured me constantly we were nearly there. The distance between Rugby and London is about 130 kilometres. But when I heard him say, 'There's the North Circular and there's our London police escort,' I knew we actually *were* nearly there since the North Circular is a ring road around Central London. The police escort that had accompanied me from Rugby was now being replaced by a police escort from London, which picked us up on the North Circular.

As we completed the last leg of the journey to the Hammersmith, I thought of the suddenness of what had just occurred. I'd been moments off crashing out in my bed and getting some shut-eye before another work day at the office in Rugby. Now, I was hurtling down the M1 motorway in the middle of the night with a police escort, not sure if I would live or die. I couldn't help but think, '*Is this it? How long have I got? Is Dr Death calling seriously this time?*'

I don't know how long the journey was, perhaps about two hours. I was fearful of another bleed and my survival instincts were on full alert; I was constantly assessing the situation. We finally arrived at the Hammersmith and I was admitted into the casualty department, which seemed quiet and relaxed. The doctor I saw was a surgeon I had met before. He arranged for me to go to Ward A8 under the care of Professor Allison, the radiologist who had carried out the previous embolisations, and told me the vascular surgeons would see me in the morning.

As I lay there in the casualty department, waiting for the doctor, I overhead a nurse say to one of her colleagues, 'What a waste of taxpayers' money – all that for one patient!' She'd seen the army entourage and police escort as I'd arrived. This shocked and appalled me, but, in my moment of rage, I still gave her the benefit of the doubt. I told myself that maybe her attitude was due to the suffering she saw every day, rather than her just being insensitive. It made me ask myself: Should they have just let me take my chances and risk death by not getting me to the Hammersmith? It was an important life lesson for me – about being sensitive to other people's feelings and not making presumptions or judgements about the actions of others. I have carried that attitude with me since that day.

CHAPTER 8

Dr Death Comes Calling

Case notes: Patient ... wants to know what can be done to stabilise maxilla/mandible. Options are 1) radical dissection including vascular, plastics and max fac 2) radical embolisation – accept loss of sight as significant risk with possible skin loss 3) surgery following embolisation. Plan 1) To get in touch with various interested surgeons who have the necessary expertise. John Lynn feels it is beyond his scope. Plan 2) Arrange admission for CT to assess AVM.

I couldn't sleep that night in Ward A8 where they'd assigned me a bed. The bedsheets were starched and stiff against my skin, and I found them irritating. However, I told myself this was probably a good sign – I was still alive and able to feel discomfort. With the nauseating stench of congealed blood in my mouth and the sweat of my body, I felt dirty, disorientated and tired. Staring out the window at the orange street lamps far off in the distance, I thought to myself, '*Life goes on and onwards we struggle – me and the patients around me, all no doubt struggling in our own way.*' The nature of things seemed clear in that environment: some of us would die, some of us would live on, and that was that.

Morning came and the night staff changed to day staff, and with them came a familiar voice. It was Noel, one of the student nurses I'd met in the summer of 1986 when I was having an embolisation procedure. I met Steve Cook at that time too – the friend who later moved to New York and whose leaving party I had meant to go to before all of this happened. He was having a small procedure back then, and I was recovering from the embolisation. We were the same age as most of the nurses and we all got on really well. Steve and I would run about on the wards in wheelchairs with these fake googly eyes hanging out of our eye sockets. We thought it was hilarious. Anyway … it was great to see Noel and reminisce a little and, of course, fill him in about my current crisis.

Within a few hours that Friday morning, though, my face began to swell even more, as if internal bleeding was occurring in the tissues. Feeling anxious and alarmed, I mentioned this to the doctors, but there were questions around what could actually be done. Professor Allison was hesitant to do further embolisations as it had not fully worked for me in the past. The thinking was that perhaps a combination of embolisation and surgery was the only hope.

Professor Allison and Miss Avril Mansfield, a vascular surgeon, initiated a call to some plastic surgeons who might be able to help. Professor Allison had previously referred a patient with a small AVM to Mr Brent Tanner, a consultant plastic surgeon at the Queen Victoria Hospital (QVH) in East Grinstead.

As time was short and the prospect of another bleed was ever present, arrangements were made for me to be transferred to the QVH. The mode of transport would be an air ambulance because of the danger of another bleed and the ongoing ambulance strike. A pilot, medic and doctor accompanied me on board for the twenty-minute journey. As I was mobile, I was able to sit up and take stock of what was going on. The helicopter took off from the carpark at the back of the hospital next to Wormwood Scrubs, and I could actually see inside the men's prison at the southern end as the ambulance elevated above it. There were also some excellent views over the River Thames and London. The pilot kindly gave me a running commentary throughout, which made the flight quite entertaining, though the occasional turbulence tickled my stomach.

As we approached the QVH, we manoeuvred and turned smoothly for a perfect landing. There was quite a crowd awaiting my arrival, including a fire engine and firemen, nurses and many other people. Apparently, they weren't used to seeing patients walking out of an air ambulance, so my arrival there seemed almost presidential.

As I walked from the helicopter, a staff nurse approached and suggested I take a seat in a wheelchair, upon which I was wheeled into the Canadian Wing, which was specifically for plastic and maxillofacial surgery patients. I was shown to my quarters – bed eighteen of forty-eight beds – situated in a bay of four beds right next to the nurses' station. A staff nurse admitted me formally with all the various bits of paperwork. It occurred to me that, in all the times I had been an in-patient, I had never been on a plastic surgery ward.

The patient in the bed next to me had his jaw wired; he was a police officer who had been involved in a local Friday night pub brawl. I wandered up and down the ward, looking at the many bizarre medical conditions of the patients. One guy in my bay was almost covered in head bandages, a moan or a grumble being his only form of communication. A male nurse was attending to him and changing his drip. I noticed the tube went into his nose and I thought, '*I hope I don't end up like that.*' Little did I know...

You could categorise the typical patients into three main conditions. Firstly, elderly people with various skin cancers; secondly, young guys who'd had motorbike accidents; and thirdly, burns victims. Most patients had muscle flaps, a technique which allows muscle from one part of the body to be connected to another part. It is somewhat shocking to look at, but an ingenious way of healing these patients' extreme injuries or burns. This technique had been pioneered at the QVH by Sir Archibald McIndoe, a plastic surgeon from New Zealand, who founded a centre for plastic and jaw surgery at the hospital to treat injured airmen of the Royal Air Force ('McIndoe's guinea pigs'), often horrifically burned during the Second World War.

~

On Monday morning, I met with Brent Tanner, the plastic surgeon, and Peter Banks, the consultant maxillofacial surgeon. As I sat in the dental chair, I studied the two surgeons with their teams, discussing the scans recently taken at the Hammersmith. They seemed excited and positively bubbling with confidence as they suggested various operating techniques such as scraping the mandible, packing the mandible and ligation (tying off) of feeder vessels. My mind wandered to the operation I'd had in 1981 when John Lynn had found collateral vessels opening up and how he'd said I would likely suffer a fatal haemorrhage if I was ever operated on again.

As I listened to Banks and Tanner discussing ideas, I realised I'd had this problem for almost a decade. What could they do that nobody else had tried? But what alternative was there? Giving up and waiting for the next bleed that might kill me? At least they were attempting to come up with a solution…

That evening, two friends from Rugby, Dusty and Nick, came to visit, and we sat in the TV lounge of the Canadian Wing. They wanted to know what my options were. I told them matter-of-factly that there were three basic options as I saw them. The first option was to do nothing, knowing and accepting that there is only one guarantee in life and that is we will all die (and of course pay taxes). Choosing this option meant death would not be long coming my way. The second option was to have a massive head and neck resection, which could lead to me losing half my face, with no real guaranteed success in solving the problem. We referred to this option as 'commando surgery' and it really did not appeal to me. The third option was to have an embolisation procedure followed by complex surgery, which seemed logical and reasonable.

Dusty and Nick stared at me in shock as I outlined these frightening options. Just by looking at them, I could tell they were thinking, '*What? This is off the Richter scale here!*' The Jerry Morrissey they'd known up to this point was a guy who enjoyed a few laughs, a few jokes, a few beers, having a good time … it must have been difficult for them to comprehend the fact that I now faced (no pun intended) such a life-or-death decision and was talking about it in such a calm and straightforward way. I think this was a coping mechanism to emotionally distance myself from the magnitude of it. However, I wasn't suppressing or avoiding any of my emotions. I allowed them to surface, but I wasn't overwhelmed by them.

'It certainly puts your everyday working problems in

perspective as rather insignificant!' exclaimed Dusty, shaking his head in disbelief.

One of the junior plastic surgeons, Per Hall, had come by and spoken to me earlier that evening. Per had a great bedside manner and a genuine approach, and I felt like I could be open with him about how I truly felt. When he left, he said he'd call by again in the morning to discuss my options further. After he left, I jotted down a few ideas in a flowchart: what my options were, the consequences and so on. It helped me to see it in a visual form like that.

The doctors had agreed I should leave the hospital the next day. They told me they would come up with a plan of action for surgery within a few weeks. The next morning I waited for Per Hall to drop by; I was really keen to discuss my ideas from the previous evening. By lunchtime, he still hadn't appeared and I learned that he'd had to go to Brighton to attend an outpatient clinic. I was disappointed, as there were so many technical questions about the procedure I wanted to ask before I left. I explained my concerns to a staff nurse who, fortuitously – though I didn't know it at the time – suggested I stay for another night so I could see the whole surgical team in the morning. I gratefully accepted.

At about six o'clock that night, my supper was delivered, and I shifted the bedside table and sat upright to eat. It was a soft meal since that's all I could manage. Yet moments later, I began to bleed inside my mouth and it quickly became uncontrollable. Within moments I realised this was the most intense bleed I had ever had. The blood was pumping out of my mouth in an almost projectile manner with every beat of my heart.

A young Irish nurse, Bridget, happened to walk past on her way to the nurses' office. I was to find out later she'd spoken to the head nurse and said, 'I didn't know they were serving beetroot on the menu tonight!' The nurse in charge, Ali, had said, 'They're not!' Bridget explained that the Scottish guy in bed eighteen was covered in what looked like beetroot. Ali looked out the office window to where I was lying. I had been placed in the bay closest to the nurses' station in case something like this happened. 'Oh, shit!' she said when she saw my big green hospital counterpane full of blood. 'Bridget – put a call out!'

It was a forty-eight-bed male plastic surgery unit and it was busy – always busy. The nurses were rushed off their feet. Ali raced out to me with a big pack of gauze and ripped it open. I grabbed a wodge and jammed it in my mouth and held it there. Ali quickly realised it was an arterial bleed and we couldn't let any pressure off.

The staff reacted immediately, wheeling me around to an anaesthetic room next to the operating theatres, where I lay losing a massive amount of blood, second by second, minute by minute.

A mass of medical people surrounded me as the clothes I was wearing were cut from me with scissors and a urine catheter inserted. I felt physically and mentally naked. I was starting to feel so cold … my hands and feet in particular. The doctors were trying to put a line in to replace some of the blood I was pumping out, but all the veins the doctors would normally stick a line into had just shut down due to the blood loss. All the remaining blood had moved to protect my vital organs from organ failure. It was as if my cells had all gone into the foetal position to protect me. The medical staff had to go for bigger vessels in the neck and groin.

Two or three times, they tried to insert a central venous pressure line directly into my heart to pump blood into my heart and major vessels. But this meant having to remove my hand from my mouth, which resulted in more bleeding. A catch-22. I could hear the heart rate monitor behind me recording my heartbeat. I told myself not to panic, even though I could hear the rapid rate of my pulse. It was a matter of survival, so I focused on using what faculties I could to control my heartbeat, regulate it and slow it down.

At one point, a doctor named Marina was reassuring me, asking me where I lived and other questions just to keep me conscious. I couldn't answer, of course, with my hand in my mouth, so I started writing things down using my left hand. At one point I even started playing a game of Hangman. I think she was shocked, if not amazed, that – given the vast quantities of blood loss – I could still be calm and rational in my behaviour. But I'd had plenty of practice at staying in control during extreme circumstances and near-death experiences. I knew what I needed to do to keep myself and those tending to me as calm as possible.

Throughout the evening, the staff asked several times if they should call my parents, who were back from Germany and staying at Stanmore Park, an air force camp in North London, a couple of hours' drive from East Grimstead on the M25. I said no each time as they would be in bed and I didn't want to disturb their sleep. Since my condition was extremely serious, they called them anyway. When they arrived, it must have looked like *The Texas Chainsaw Massacre* in that ante-theatre. It wouldn't have been a vision they were likely to forget either – their son lying saturated in his own blood, hooked up to all kinds of lines and tubes, as close to death as they had ever seen him.

After they left, a consultant anaesthetist suggested I have a jab in the wrist. I was afraid they were planning the commando-style surgery that had been discussed, where they would go in and ligate all the big feeder vessels – almost take my face off, like a battlefield casualty, and do whatever it took, chopping away at everything. It was an emphatic 'NO' from me. I wrote down, 'Just get me to the Hammersmith again!' I knew I needed an embolisation to get the bleeding under control. Once the blood flow was not as aggressive and not pumping out, a major operation could be done … but with more control than the commando surgery. I felt in my heart the latter would kill me or render me a vegetable. I was also quite prepared to do nothing and risk bleeding to death. Even that seemed preferable to the commando surgery.

At this point, I wanted to get to the Hammersmith as soon as possible, so I wrote this down again for the surgical staff, and Brent Tanner agreed to contact Professor Allison. He was at home since it was late evening by then. However, when Mr Tanner explained my predicament, Professor Allison agreed that an immediate embolisation should be carried out. He said he would call out his team and operate on me through the night.

After many hours of being jammed in my mouth, my right arm became completely numb. I had to concentrate and continually force myself mentally to 'pitch in there'. After four hours, I let my hand out while Ali tried to stop the blood, but it was to no avail; it continued to pump out all over me, covering the bed and the floor. Measuring jugs were used to estimate the blood loss, but so much had soaked through the sheets and blankets that it was impossible to calculate. With so little blood in my body, I was getting closer to death. Per Hall tried to stop the blood. 'Just give me a chance, Jerry,' he said. I did, and he struggled inside my mouth until I could take no more, and I forced his hand out and mine back in.

Panic consumed me, driven by the fear of the unknown and the impending, inevitable end. Despite a desperate survival instinct, I grappled with the harsh reality that the situation was beyond my or the surgical team's control. With each beat of my heart, blood pumped out of my body and my strength ebbed away, accompanied by dizziness and a chilling coldness as blood loss escalated. This physical deterioration paralleled a profound emotional experience – feelings of isolation and loneliness, and a stark confrontation with my own mortality.

This harrowing experience stripped away any illusions of control, leaving me to face the bare truth that no one was coming to save me. Then, amid the chaos, a curious serenity washed over me as acceptance of my fate settled in. My struggle waned, replaced by an eerie tranquillity, a strange comfort in the face of the inevitable. I found an odd peace, almost a readiness to embrace the end of my life.

It seemed as if my life fluid was draining away from me. And as it did so, my whole life played out in front of me in fast-forward mode, just as they say it does at the end of life: being a baby, pre-school, all the places I had ever been to and the people I had met … and with this series of flashbacks, Dr Death truly seemed to be calling my name this time.

It was all too much for my body so was then a case of lights out.

~

Case notes: Per Hall (Plastics) to Mr Smith (Cardio). Bleed 5 litres and emergency transfer to Hammersmith in the middle of the night.

Case report: Following a life-threatening alveolar haemorrhage in February 1990, from which he nearly exsanguinated, he was resuscitated and then underwent successful emergency embolisation.

With time being of the essence, an air ambulance would have to be called, but the air ambulance wasn't operational that evening because of high winds and bad weather. The only other hope was to call in the Royal Air Force. More special treatment from the armed forces ... hopefully the same nurse who couldn't believe 'all this for one man' wouldn't be on emergency when we arrived at the Hammersmith this time.

By that stage, the bleeding had slowed and eventually stopped. By then, nurse Ali had her hand in my mouth, applying pressure to stop the bleeding, as I'd been in and out of consciousness. Eventually, I stabilised sufficiently for her to take her hand out of my mouth and I was all packed up, ready for the transfer to the Hammersmith.

As the RAF helicopter arrived, hovering above the helipad outside the burns unit, the aircrew took control and organised the transfer swiftly and efficiently. As I lay there steeped in blood, I looked up and saw this large handle-bar moustache. It belonged to one of the aircrew who calmly and assertively gave orders to everyone, ensuring each person knew what was required of them. It was go, go, go until we got up in the air and on our way. The consultant anaesthetist, Keith Judkins, Ali and an operating technician were on the flight as well.

The sheer size and power of the Sea King helicopter meant it certainly wasn't a comfortable experience. As we flew above East Grinstead, it was incredibly noisy. The blood-soaked gauze still positioned along the contours inside my mouth didn't move for the entire journey. My face, body and mind were numb. They'd sedated me to keep me stable throughout the trip, so I didn't wake bolt upright going, 'Woah, where am I?' Obviously, that could easily lead to blood spurting out all over again. But I must have been in and out of consciousness because I could hear Ali asking, 'Jerry, can you hear me? Can you hear me?' I was also aware of her taking my blood pressure every now and again.

I travelled that journey a very lonely man. I was locked on one thing: SURVIVAL. This was it – a desperate last-ditch attempt to save my life. Embolisation at the Hammersmith followed by possible surgery at the QVH – if I did not bleed to death in the meantime.

It must have been incredibly intense for Ali and Keith, waiting to fly into action at any moment. They were fully expecting more spurts of blood once we got into the air, so they had all kinds of medical paraphernalia ready to go, just in case.

Fortunately, that did not happen. As the chopper came in to land, a sea of white coats awaited us. I was transferred to a trolley and wheeled across the tarmac. Medical staff were wheeling intravenous poles and oxygen equipment, and it was noisy, rattly and windy. We finally made it into the Hammersmith and inside the lift. I was vaguely aware that Keith and Ali were still with me, along with the Hammersmith staff. There were so many people pushing the trolley along and holding drips and other bits and pieces that it was quite squashed in the lift.

One of the Hammersmith staff was explaining that the theatre was prepped and ready to go for the embolisation. As the lift stopped and the doors opened, some kind of kerfuffle ensued. I could hear exclamations and swearing. I learned later that the lift had stopped several inches short of the floor for some inexplicable reason. All the staff surrounding me pitched in to lift the trolley and someone counted '1, 2, 3, go' as they hoisted me out of the lift. It must have been a very surreal moment for all of them but I don't recall that part of the proceedings!

Clink, clink, clink, down the corridor we went. They wheeled me into a theatre prep room and there was something of a briefing and handover, after which Ali and Keith left.

Professor Allison and the surgical team were ready, preparing for the embolisation. I was unable to move my head because further bleeding could result, so a gentle nod was my only form of communication with them. A nurse began shaving my thigh and groin hair and applying antiseptic to the area, preparing for the groin puncture into the femoral artery.

The procedure started with Professor Allison pushing the catheter in, which would then be pushed up through my abdomen and heart, and into my head and neck. The x-ray machine that followed the wire was only a few centimetres above my face and connected to a video display unit so the professor could direct the catheter where it needed to go. I could feel the wire as it entered my head.

I was gazing up, looking at all the vessels the injected dye would highlight, when, without warning, the screen went blank. The machine had stopped working and we couldn't continue. I couldn't believe it – what next? As the staff checked out the machine, I lay there thinking, '*Why the hell isn't this bloody machine working?*' My heart was sinking; yet another layer of mental torture was weighing me down even further.

There were two angiography theatres at the Hammersmith: the one we were in with the all-singing, all-dancing machine; and the other next door – a capable but bog-standard version. The only thing for it was to transfer next door, which meant pulling the wire out of my body and having to re-insert it all over again in the new room. It was devastating for me, but necessary.

The team inserted another wire and there was a strong feeling of warmth in my head and neck as the dye was injected. The professor could then see which feeder arteries he wanted to block off and where he wanted to inject the spring coils. I could feel every coil turn and twist into position in my head. As more coils went in, the pain became even more intense.

Being fully awake without general anaesthesia amplified the torment, transforming the pain into a vicious onslaught of sharp, intense stabbing sensations that contorted my body in a frenzy of agony. Each passing second dragged on like an eternity, every moment an anguished plea for relief. The pain reverberated through me, leaving me gasping for air as beads of sweat dripped from every pore of my body, a physical manifestation of the overwhelming fear and anguish I felt. For the love of God, could this pain just stop! It was a hellish nightmare with no escape. The whole procedure took a few hours, and the professor blocked as many vessels as he could, reducing the blood flow rate.

But once he was done, what would the next step be? It was three or four o'clock in the morning, and Professor Allison thought I should return to the QVH immediately. If I started to bleed again, he said no more could be done for me and I would certainly just bleed to death. Only the dreaded commando surgery at the QVH would then offer any hope. It would be just a few hours until daybreak when the air ambulance started operating. The young doctor working alongside Professor Allison suggested we wait until then as it would be more comfortable and safer than relying on some other form of transport. After some debate between the professor and the young doctor, it was decided we would wait until morning.

I spent the next few hours in a ward, my mind disorientated and hazy. I was vomiting constantly and couldn't help but wonder if I would still be alive to see the sun rise. Physically wrecked and mentally pushed to the limit, my body was running on reserve energy. I dozed on and off until they came to collect me for the helicopter journey back to the QVH.

This time I did not see any of the flight. I was horizontal and full of intravenous drips, and so exhausted that I was finally able to feel some strange level of relaxation. Perhaps the daylight hours had brought back some level of hope for me … and where there is life there is hope … right?

~

Meanwhile, back at the QVH, the staff who'd taken care of me during the bleed had all gone to the bar in the doctors' mess for a drink, needing to unwind after the trauma of dealing with me. The next morning they were all hungover, probably still fast asleep, when they got beeped or buzzed to say the patient was coming back from the Hammersmith. Panic ensued as they got up in a hurry to meet the air ambulance and get me into the intensive care ward. They certainly didn't expect me to be coming back so soon.

Ali remembers staying up all night after she got back about 4am. The operating department assistants had been cleaning up my blood, which was all over the ante-theatre. As she was on an early shift the next day, she stayed at work, thinking there was no point in sleeping as she was still buzzing from the adrenaline. One of the operating department assistants took her outside for a fag, even though she didn't smoke, until her shift started at 7am.

It was the talk of the hospital, afterwards – 'Did you hear about what happened?' – since it was only a small hospital and everybody knew each other. The joke of it was that Ali got in trouble for her part in helping save my life. Her unit manager pulled her aside, and Ali thought she was about to be congratulated. Instead, she received a bollocking because she'd left the ward unattended without a senior nurse.

Even now, all these years later, Ali still can't believe the unfairness of that!

CHAPTER 9

Decision Time

Case notes: Treated recently by embolisation by Prof Allison. Massive blood transfusion/embolisation. Admitted for consideration of excision of AVM under by-pass conditions.

Back at the QVH, I did not return to the Canadian Wing but to the Russell Davies Unit (RDU), a mini intensive care unit, and had one-on-one nursing for the next week. For the first few days, I just slept. My dietary intake consisted of three baby beakers of 'food' – one soup, one soft meat and the other a milkshake known as 'liquid jaw', usually given to patients with wired jaws. Once again, I felt relaxed in a strange sort of way – though with hindsight it must have been the drugs they were pumping into me. I honestly thought things could not get worse. How wrong could I be?

The surgeons breezed in and out, discussing and debating what could be done. The key problem was that my AVM was so large and, under arterial pressure, the blood just pumped out, which made surgery a very tricky prospect. Nick Parkhouse was a senior registrar in plastic surgery who came up with a really out-there suggestion: let's temporarily kill Jerry to give us a time window to operate, then start him back up again.

WTF was this guy on? He was a flamboyant, larger-than-life character who would often fly above the hospital in his Tiger Moth. He had a crazy, creative mind – maybe he was onto something? But what did he mean by killing me and bringing me back to life? Did he think he was Jesus, and I some sort of biblical Lazarus character?

His theory was that they would carry out a heart-lung bypass on me. They would disconnect my heart and lungs from my body and connect my main arteries to a heart-lung machine. This would enable them to control the blood flow through the body and brain, and keep a sufficiency of blood flowing to keep me alive. It would also give them time to operate on the AVM. They would make an incision from ear to ear, lift back my skin like a face mask, ligate all the feeder vessels, remove all the lower teeth, inject me with a solution called STD (a gluing agent used in the treatment of varicose veins) and rebuild my jaw by using part of my pelvis (iliac crest), which they would remove for that purpose.

Rightio! It sounded like I was going to be opened up all over – heart, lungs, hip, face … would I really be able to survive that?

The medical staff and my parents, when they were informed, were convinced this was the only chance. I was not so sure. Over the next couple of days in the RDU, I slept on and off. I was still weak and somewhat vague about what was going on around me because of the blood loss and trauma I'd been through. I tried to take in the gist of the conversations I could hear going on around me.

Instinctively I felt this operation would fail. What that meant I wasn't sure, but, if nothing was done, I would certainly bleed to death within a few weeks. What a choice! I wanted to make certain I had all the facts and feel confident in my decision. However, lying on the bed, hearing only half sentences exchanged between my parents and the surgeons, I struggled to join in.

My mother, it seemed, had found the flowchart I had made the day before my near fatal bleed. It was basically a brainstorming session with myself – the plusses and minuses, pros and cons, working it all through in my head. Only my mother's interpretation was completely different to mine – she seemed to think I was all for this operation and she was setting the wheels in motion for it to go ahead. I tried in vain to explain: 'No, no, no! I don't mean that!' But my exhaustive state from the embolisation rendered me unable to think in any rational or logical way. I wanted some time to reach a conclusion on my own so that, whatever happened, I knew I'd made the choice myself. It was my life. Whether I died or was paralysed, I was the one who had to live with the choice I made.

But this unprecedented, monumental procedure – involving killing me, no less – was already being accepted as a feasible, practical operation and it was already being planned without my go-ahead. In fact, they'd already set a date. It was to be carried out at the Hammersmith on Friday, 2 March 1990, only two days after the embolisation. To my relief, it was cancelled since my blood platelet level was way too low.

That gave me a few days' grace to make up my mind. In the meantime, the maxillofacial and plastic surgeons from the QVH were discussing it all with the Hammersmith doctors. Professor Allison had contacted Mr Smith, a consultant heart surgeon at the Hammersmith. His team could fit me in for Thursday, 8 March 1990, allocating a full day in the operating theatre at the

Criteria/ Options	1. Do nothing	2. Embolisation(s) then surgery	3. Radical surgery with heart/lung bypass
Likelihood of surviving the operation?	• Not Applicable. Leave AVM as is.	• Low/Medium – risk of brain damage, loss of sight. Survived this combination before.	• Very Low – effectively taking my head from my body and opening my chest.
Probability of successfully removing the AVM?	• No change. If anything, the AVM will get larger by doing nothing.	• Low – been tried before. At best the AVM will reduce in size for a period of time.	• Medium/High – would give the best surgical approach to removing the AVM.
Quality of life: post-operation.	• Continue 'as is' with a poor quality of life.	• At best quality of life stays 'as is' or potential for brain damage.	• Totally unknown. If I do survive, could end up with severe brain damage, in a wheelchair.

EMERGING THOUGHTS FROM OPTION ANALYSIS (RISK V BENEFIT):

Option 1: This option guarantees bleeding to death, which will most likely occur within days or weeks.

Option 2: This option has been done before. It delays the inevitable, providing more time alive (months) but resulting in poor quality of life. It involves a slow, painful existence until a fatal bleed.

Option 3: This would be a medical first, involving a combination of surgical techniques not done before. If I die, it is likely to happen on the operating table, so I will feel no pain and have no concept of ever being alive. From a first-principles point of view, theoretically, it might work to remove the AVM.

DECISION:

Option 3: This is the only option that could successfully remove the life-threatening condition. However, the probability of surviving the operation is low (though it will be a painless death if it occurs on the operating table). If I do survive, I may be paralysed, severely brain-damaged, have limited mobility, and so on. The road to recovery will be long and complicated. If I decide on Option 3, I will need to fully accept and live with the consequences of my post-operative condition, whatever that may be.

Options Analysis: What should I do?

1. Do Nothing
2. Embolisation(s) then surgery
3. Radical surgery with heart/ lung bypass

Hammersmith with the surgical team from the QVH travelling up from Sussex.

I continued to have an internal debate on whether to have this previously untried combination of operating techniques done all at once. The operation would offer some chance, whereas no operation would mean certain death. I had my reasons for considering both options.

I was thinking of the future if I had the operation – what my future state might be. I didn't want to die, but it was a reality I might not wake up. And if I did, I could wake up paralysed or having had a stroke. I could end up a vegetable. Did I want to survive if that was the case?

We are constantly faced with decisions as we navigate our way through life. And there are always consequences, good or bad. When a decision is made, you must live with these consequences. It was therefore of paramount importance to me to make the decision myself based on as much information as I could get. I knew if I was 'lucky' enough to survive the operation, I would have to live in the 'real' world even if I was horribly disfigured or immobile in a wheelchair.

After much inner debate, I decided 'yes'. I was prepared to live with the consequences – whatever they may be. It was family and friends who helped me make the decision to have the operation – their presence in my life certainly boosted any inherent survival instinct I had, and I thank them for that. It's a powerful quality and one that I admire in people – doing things for others, or simply being there, and not expecting anything in return. A rare and commendable quality.

Once the decision was made, I remained in the RDU, trying to make the most of my time before the mega-operation and its outcome. Phone calls from family and friends were frequent. In fact, they became so common the nurse detached the phone from the wall and put it beside my bed.

I had a steady stream of visitors too. My good friend Mark, whom I'd met in Germany, and his long-term partner Julie came to visit, which was a highlight for me during that time. They were off to live and work in Italy, but they made the effort to come and see me. I also had a visit from Tom Richardson from GEC, which was most welcome.

The nurses were of great comfort to me as well. My night nurse, Vicky, had a wicked sense of humour and was constantly threatening to pull the urine catheter out of my body if I misbehaved, which made me squirm. Or she would make certain threats about the bottom (rectal) thermometer they had inserted, which was so bloody uncomfortable that I repeatedly removed it. It measured my core body temperature and was connected to a digital output device that compared it with my peripheral temperature (via a device placed on my big toe). Tremendous, eh? Just what you needed in a weak, uncomfortable state when your only comfort was to balance your body weight on the right or left butt cheek.

My day nurse, Liz, usually worked in the burns unit of the hospital. She had the ignominious job of lancing all the zits on my face. I had awoken one morning to find my face covered in zits. Had the spot fairy visited overnight? No, apparently it was the antibiotics and nervous strain on my body producing them. Liz actually seemed to delight in the successful lancing and removal of them, so I was glad I could oblige.

One thing I did learn: there is no room for any embarrassment when your physical body is exposed to all on a daily basis –

whether it be a thermometer being shoved up your ass, a catheter stuck up your urethra, a bed bath, someone wiping your bum after you've shat the bed, insertion and removal of the bedpan … I could go on. The indignity of such bodily functions disappears when you realise survival is the main issue – your *life* is the main issue. Such bodily functions are normal and natural, and you just have to crack on with it. No room for red faces.

In readiness for the operation, I conditioned myself physically and mentally. Once I'd made up my mind, mentally preparing was easier as I'd already come to terms with the possible consequences. But physically, I needed to build up my strength because they wouldn't operate unless my blood platelets were up and everything had stabilised, so I continued to take in as much food as I could from my baby beakers. Solid food wasn't an option since further bleeding could mean the end, full stop.

On Tuesday, 6 March 1990, I flew out again by helicopter to the Hammersmith to get ready for the operation.

The day before the operation was hectic. More friends, relations and close family visited, and the phone calls continued, making every minute extremely valuable for me. Again, I reflected on how privileged I was to have such a wonderful family and caring friends. During the day, I took them between the TV room of Ward A8 and my bed as I discussed my operation. I was very aware of the fact that it was perhaps the last time they were seeing me as a functional human being.

During my stay at the Russell Davies Unit at the QVH, after creating my option analysis of which medical approach I should take, I made a pivotal decision: I would take full responsibility for whatever condition I emerged in after the operation. If the surgeons had made that decision for me, I might have been bitter or resentful if I had ended up paralysed and in a wheelchair. However, by making the decision myself, I would embrace the outcome and confront reality head-on.

I spoke to Professor Hall, an anaesthetist, and Mr Smith, the consultant heart surgeon. They explained their particular 'bits' of the operation, since state-of-the-art technologies and complex surgical techniques – in maxillofacial, plastics, heart, anaesthesia and radiology – were all coming together for this one operation. Mr Smith pointed out he'd be doing an operation on a healthy heart, a concept he seemed quite taken by, since heart surgeons don't usually do operations on healthy hearts. But he did tell me about what could go wrong – that I could die or have a stroke – though the plastic surgeons tried to be a bit more upbeat about it.

Professor Allison came to see me while some friends were visiting. 'This is your only real chance of survival,' he said, pointing out that while something bad could happen, 'the alternative is that you bleed to death – that's a guarantee.' He also added that it was an operation so radical in nature it would be the first time such a combination of surgical techniques had been used all at once. My friends' jaws were basically on the ground when they heard about the immensity of what I was facing.

Later that evening, I had a visit from Adrienne – a fellow member of the Gruesome Foursome. We took a trip down memory lane remembering the previous summer, drinking vast amounts of alcohol together and travelling around in the Mobile Coffin. She fondly called me 'Jeremiah Obediah' since we all had daft nicknames for each other. Richard was Mr Bloody Immature because he always acted like a daft kid. Adrienne was Aids because it was simple just to shorten her name. Sarah was known as Hue-mung-guy Butt-eye, which means 'extremely large, fat bottom'. She didn't have one, but the fact that this name irritated her immensely provided great entertainment and mirth for the rest of us. It was fun to just relax a little with Adrienne and recall the good times, considering what might happen in the next twenty-four hours.

A little later, Rachel Beirne arrived. Rachel was a nurse at the Hammersmith, and she and I had known each other back in 1986 when I was an in-patient in Ward D1. She was wild, with a bizarre hairdo in those days. She reminded me of a sad occasion on D1 all those years ago, a rare time when I was close to tears.

D1 was a ward full of patients with liver and bladder issues. One patient was a Scotsman, James, who had liver cancer. He seemed like a genuine type of bloke and I met his family. He had his operation and was placed in Ward D2 for high dependency patients. I visited him a few days after his operation and spoke to him in my usual friendly manner. He didn't recognise me, despite our chats prior to the operation.

'Who are you?' he asked. He began to pull the tubes from his stomach and bladder. 'I don't want these,' he shouted. I stood there in my pyjamas and looked into his eyes. His mind was bewildered, illogical. What the hell had happened to him? His liver was the problem, not his mind.

As I entered D1, Rachel had seen me looking disturbed. 'What's the matter, Jerry?' she said. I explained what had happened with James. She told me that although the liver can regenerate a certain amount, if too much is removed through surgery, the poisons in the body cannot be broken down and travel through the blood system to the brain – hence his present mental condition. A few days later, he died. I lay on my bed that night and thought not only of his death but of his life, his family and his children.

I also thought of his life and death mathematically for some reason:

- at a time t = -1 second, alive;
- at a time t = 0, dying; and
- at a time t = +1 second, dead.

At the point of t = +1 second, all of the knowledge and all of the experiences of one individual were gone, forever.

Rachel, a real chatterbox, was talking away while Adrienne listened, or perhaps she was further reflecting on times gone by. I was pleased they had both come to visit. Adrienne had also sent a card and flowers, and called several times, which was sweet of her since we had not seen each other for months. '*I'm going to miss her,*' I thought. '*I might never see her again.*' She left around 11pm and Rachel shortly after.

At midnight, I bathed and shaved all my body hair from the groin upwards, and took the pre-operation pills. I was already stained on the face and chest with a brown iodine-type substance in readiness for the next day. Considering the major operation I was facing, I slept surprisingly well.

At 7am on Thursday, 8 March 1990, I went off to the operating theatre, thinking, '*Here we go … today could be the last day of my life.*'

CHAPTER 10

Killing Jerry

Case report: ... underwent surgery after establishing extracorporeal bypass circulation. The intramandibular portion of the malformation was treated by complete lower dental clearance and packing of the curetted medullary cavity with methylmethacrylate cement and iliac crest bone graft. Intratumoral ligation sutures were then placed into the facial and neck segments of the malformation and STD sclerosant injections were also given.

Professor Allison told me later he had come into the operating theatre during the procedure and was shocked: it looked like a post-mortem was being undertaken. My chest cavity had been cut open and the ribcage spread apart. My heart had been stopped and connected to a heart-lung bypass machine. I'd had a tracheotomy so a breathing tube connected to a ventilator could be placed in my lungs through a hole in my throat. My face had been pulled back so they could access my jaw, which had been dislocated in order for them to remove the teeth one by one and perform the surgery on the mandible. This involved scraping out the AVM itself, which was soft and spongey, then plugging up the holes in the area with chips of bone from my hip, which had been opened up for the bone extraction. Professor Allison said at that point he questioned whether it was really worth putting me through all this … had they made the right decision or was it just an outrageous idea that would backfire?

Colin Hopper, the maxillofacial surgeon from East Grinstead who removed my teeth, also told me later that he was left holding my mandible while the rest of the team went off for a cup of tea in the middle of the operation… I must say this was rather shocking to hear!

The operation took place on a Thursday and lasted eleven or twelve hours. I only started to regain consciousness on the Saturday afternoon.

But before I did, I had this strange out-of-body experience. I was in that dreamy half-awake, half-asleep state when this woman appeared and told me her name was Amanda. I was trying to get up – but it would have been impossible for me to get up in the state I was in. She put her hand on my chest and said, 'It's not your time,' and milliseconds later I became consciously aware of where I was – in the Hammersmith. It seemed so real, but then our dreams often do. Some might also say it was the anaesthetic wearing off and that being out of it for so long can make your brain play funny tricks on you. All of that may be true, but what sticks with me most is this woman saying, 'It's not your time' – and I guess it wasn't. But surviving is one thing … thriving is something else entirely.

Case notes (10/03/1990): 5pm awake and orientated. Unable to open eyes.

Those early hours and days were all a bit hazy to me. I was told that, as I was beginning to regain consciousness, I had been put into an induced coma so my body would tolerate being on the ventilator, since the machine breathes for you. If you are not heavily sedated, your body will fight against the machine. When I did regain consciousness, my first contact with the living world was through the sense of hearing. I felt as if I had no physical body at all and only my mental capacities remained, which I told myself was probably the effects of the drugs numbing my body.

'Jerry, do you know where you are?' said a male voice.

Everything was so dark. With my left hand I touched my eyes. *Why couldn't I see him … or anything for that matter?* I tried nodding in answer to his question, though moving my head was almost impossible. I lifted my left hand instead.

'You're in ICU, Jerry,' said the male voice.

I don't remember anything much at all on that first day other than being aware of sounds and movement around me and the different smells of the hospital. My mother and George must've been there because I could hear their voices at one stage too.

Case notes (11/03/1990): Transient neuro disturbances.

On the Sunday, Colin Hopper arrived with a colleague. He removed the pads that were squeezed into my mouth. I was deeply concerned another bleed would occur, but Colin reassured me he'd 'removed the life-threatening condition' – that is, the AVM.

The dates and times of various events that took place over those first few days all seem fused together in my traumatised state. I heard many conversations, though I couldn't do much more than listen. One between George and an ICU nurse sticks in my mind: I could hear music in the background and the nurse asked George what sort of music I liked. In my mind, I began grasping with this question and, in my vague mental state, I managed to write down Deacon Red and Simply Blue, instead of Deacon Blue and Simply Red.

As the days went on in intensive care, I still couldn't see and I couldn't move the right side of my body. I couldn't speak because of the tracheotomy and hole in my throat, which would take weeks to heal.

> **Case notes (11/03/1990):** Paralysis has been noted on right hand side but difficult to assess. Is it due to embolic material carried down into the brain or bleed because of anti-coagulant and hypertension or residual effect of the bypass. If a clot has formed then thinning the blood would be fraught with danger.

My eyes were still closed, and the surgeons and neurologist were at a loss as to why several of my cranial nerves were apparently damaged, leading to weakness on my right-hand side. That's when they realised, at some point in the proceedings, I'd had a stroke. And that's when they also said they didn't actually know how it was all going to play out – to what level I would recover … or whether I would recover at all.

Hearing about my stroke made me feel immensely vulnerable and fearful of the unknown. Questions about the severity of the stroke, its effects on my daily life, and the path to recovery (if there was one) swirled endlessly in my mind. However, I could not ask anyone these questions because I could not speak. Anxiety gripped me as I thought about potential disabilities, leading to huge uncertainty about my future and how it would unfold. I was also worried about the burden this would place on my mum and George.

The surgeon's rule of thumb for stroke patients was based on the law of diminishing returns. You'd get the best response within a year; thereafter, it would be maybe small, incremental changes. So that was the prognosis for me. Then they said once I left intensive care at the Hammersmith, I'd need rehabilitation. Lots of rehabilitation. And the plastic surgeon wanted to tidy my face up as well.

The neurologist pulled, pushed and probed my body to assess the full extent of my physical capability. Over the next few days, he cajoled me into responding to his demanding requests. Pulling my eyelids up, he shone a torch in my eyes and asked me to move my pupils around. He moved my fingers, hand, arm and leg in what seemed like every conceivable way you could possibly imagine. I could hear his assertive voice with its Geordie accent calling out, 'Come on, Jerry lad. Come on, Jerry,' as I struggled to follow his orders. At times I just wanted to sleep, as I was completely exhausted. His encouragement did give me the strength to persevere though.

The doctors then did some MRI scans to suss out what was going on. They found two clots on the brain – one had caused the stroke and the paralysis on the right-hand side of my body: the right arm, the right leg, the right side of the tongue, both eyelids, the whole of the right body. The other, I was to find out later, left me with epilepsy.

~

On Monday evening I was moved to the high dependency ward and my left eye started to partially open. To my relief, I could identify and see images, albeit blurred.

It was at that stage I noticed the compression garment I was wearing. It fit tightly around my head and was designed to keep the tissues in place that had been cut open during the surgery, as well as reduce swelling and bruising. But with the painkillers being slightly reduced in strength, a few days after the operation I became aware of how much pain I was in and how uncomfortable the compression garment was. The time period from when a dosage began to wear off and the injection of another was most painful. My whole body was a pain-zone. The bandaged hip, chest, neck, head and mouth all seemed to be superimposed with an excruciating 'constructive wave flow' of pain. And bone pain breaks through the pain barrier – no painkillers could really get rid of the pain in my jaw, chest and hip.

The pressure garment, which someone told me later looked as if it had been made from a bra cup, was so tight around my neck it felt as if my head would explode. It was beyond the point of irritation and I could stand it no longer. I tried to take it off but the male nurse was adamant it should stay on. This debate continued, with me in a groaning manner outlining my need to remove the garment. He then called the ICU nurse who was about to leave the ward. The ICU nurse had a small bottle of Entonox. Perhaps they thought that by administering a large dose of this drug I would become unconscious and therefore they would be able to keep the pressure garment on my head. This didn't happen, however, and the loud groans and frightened movements of my body must have indicated that I was not a happy Hector. So, with the garment still on, the two nurses began to settle me into the ward.

My body wasn't having a bar of it though. Before I knew it, I was vomiting up blood. My body was riddled with spasms in an almost rhythmic fashion, each convulsion sending out a torrent of blood. A nurse tried to do a groin puncture – I have no idea why. Perhaps she thought I had an AVM in the stomach and was injecting me in readiness for an embolisation procedure. Whatever the reason, in a state of panic, she missed the target site, and the needle hit my groin. Then I could feel blood in my groin area. Pain on pain becomes intolerable and you just want it to end.

Like the many sessions of bleeding from my mouth, I soon lay steeped in my own blood. The pressure garment had come off as it was saturated in blood – a blessing in disguise for me. The next few hours were full of confusion. '*What the fuck's going on here?*' I was thinking. '*What's happening to me?*' But soon I was lapsing in and out of consciousness. No one knew if the blood loss was due to the heart-lung bypass or if I was bleeding from the stomach due to the stress of the operation. I wasn't able to eat at that point and was hooked up to a drip to get water through my arm. Perhaps I was just throwing up my stomach lining due to an ulcer from the stress of it all. No one knew, and, in the end, no surgical action took place.

That night I lay on a trolley at the end of a long corridor outside the operating theatre, not in a bed or a ward. Feeling desperately lonely, in great pain and concerned for my wellbeing, I struggled mentally throughout the entire night.

~

The morphine-based painkillers were giving me horrendous nightmares. Even in my sleep, I was haunted by terrorising scenes of bleeding to death. Dreams of bleeding from the mouth. Dreams of bleeding from the hip where they had taken the bone. A rubber tube had been inserted to drain the blood away into a little bag on the side of my hip. I dreamed that it burst and I was bleeding to death.

Then there was the night when I woke up and found there *was* blood all over the bed. The bag had burst. Those dreams were just so real – to find out it was actually happening, and to feel and smell the blood, was horrendous. Those dreams went on for years and years.

The pain was constant and my body was screaming in those first few days. I couldn't take it anymore. I decided a lethal injection would be the solution; it would be painless, like going into a deep sleep. A little injection to take all the pain away.

It was a bit like one of those challenges on *Survivor* – where the contestants are pitted against each other in some sort of gruelling challenge to see who can outlast all the rest. Say, hanging from a bar, like in the gym. You can only hang for so long. After a few minutes, everything starts to ache and then it becomes a mental battle. At some point, you have to let go because you just cannot hang there any longer. I was at that point where I just had to let go…

I told my mother when she came to visit. I wrote down: 'Just give me a lethal injection.' I don't remember her response, but years later I was talking about it to my younger brother, Paul. He told me Mum had left the hospital crying, as she had done on so many occasions. It must have been terrible for her to read those words from her child and not be able to take the pain away… She wasn't able to do *anything* really, other than be there and bear witness to the pain.

~

Case report: Postoperatively … recovery was complicated by transient brain stem ischaemia and cranial nerve dysfunction, particularly affecting the third and fourth cranial nerves; perioperative hypotension and extracorporeal bypass circulation were considered to be the most likely cause for these sequelae. A small area of superficial soft-tissue necrosis developed on the chin which was managed conservatively.

To add to my woes, with my cranial nerves not functioning properly, saliva was pooling in my lungs, which led me to cough up phlegm constantly. During the night, I would lie there with piles of tissues my parents had folded up neatly during the day.

Every few minutes, I would use a tissue. Not really conducive to good sleep. On the plus side, though, I was moved to a side room, since the bright lights of the main ward hurt my left eye as I strained to see what was going on around me.

Eating was a no-go for me as well, as it would end up with food being expelled from the hole in my throat from the tracheotomy. Intravenous drips supplied me with nutrients, but they had to be removed when they gave me a CT scan. With no fluid intake during the scan, I started rapidly dehydrating and was on the verge of collapsing. The doctor then suggested I have a naso-gastric tube for my food intake instead. The feed drip would be set at a low rate and gradually increased.

If the naso-gastric tube came out of my nose for whatever reason, a doctor was required to re-insert it. On one occasion, soon after it was inserted, I had this strange feeling – as if I was drowning. I mentioned this several times to the duty doctor, but he seemed unconcerned and suggested I relax and be a little more patient.

Some hours went by and I felt progressively worse, so I took it upon myself to switch the automatic drip feed off. I was convinced it was this that was causing the discomfort. This got the doctor's attention, and he called for a mobile x-ray machine. They wheeled it into the room and hovered it over my body. *Click, click.* Sure enough, I was right. They had actually inserted the naso-gastric tube into my lungs and not my stomach. I was slowly drowning in my food, choking to death.

Later that evening, the tube came out again and at around 10pm the nurse called the duty doctor to re-insert it. He suggested I wait until the following day, which was a decision that did not sit well with me. I knew my physical state was such that, without any nutrients, my condition would likely deteriorate even further. I didn't sleep that night. I was thoroughly pissed off, dehydrated and overheating in my bed. What I would have given for a cool bath.

The next morning, the cardiac surgeon visited me on his ward round. I was under the care of the heart surgeons who would give the all-clear once I was stabilised to return to the QVH to begin my rehabilitation. As far as the cardiac surgeons were concerned, their bit of the operation had been a success since there had been no problems with the heart-lung bypass.

A large group of neurologists then came to visit me. They probed, observed and generally made comments about my condition among themselves rather than to me. And the outcome I was hearing was not optimistic. There was no guarantee the right eyelid would open. There was no guarantee I would ever see again on that side. Right-side weakness was evident since I couldn't move my arm or leg. There was a possibility I wouldn't be able to speak again once the tracheotomy was removed. There would be balance and coordination issues due to nerve damage.

Their prognosis? Time combined with arduous physiotherapy would improve the situation. The fact that I was young (just twenty-five years old) would improve my chances of recovery. After that, they finally thought to ask me how I felt about this. Two thoughts occurred in parallel: '*I am completely pissed off*' and '*I WILL recover from this*.'

A little later, I was woken by a first-year nursing student who was there to give me a bed bath. Following the neurologists' assessment earlier that day, I just wanted to be left alone in my freakish misery. I didn't feel like doing anything. I felt like half a person and I really wanted some time inside my own mind to get my act together. The nurse was unaware of what had taken place during the ward round. She bathed me, tidied me up and put a comb in my right hand. I tried to move my hand towards my head to comb my hair, but I couldn't do it. The nurse was unaware of my screaming inner mind and I couldn't tell her even if I'd wanted to verbalise that internal rage. I wanted to be left alone to indulge myself in a good ol' dose of self-pity.

That afternoon, Jackie, the physio, came to see me. She explained that many months, if not years, of physiotherapy were ahead of me. My initial thinking was, '*Well, okay, let's start at the beginning and build my strength and bodily movements.*' I suggested a walking frame might be useful to keep my balance. Jackie said a walking stick would be alright, with her to lean on if I was feeling dodgy.

I immediately thought of myself, a twenty-five-year-old guy, walking around the streets with a walking stick, perhaps with one of those fedora hats the old boys wear. '*No, no, no,*' I thought. '*I don't need anything.*' I wrote down for Jackie that as a challenge I would walk from my bed to the toilet (and empty my urine bottle) some ten metres away and I would use her to balance on if needed (hopefully not spilling urine on her). She gently positioned my body to sit upright with my legs hanging from the bed. I stood up, disorientated but with a clear aim of the task ahead.

With all my energy focused on forward movement, I walked like a man who had consumed too many beers. I staggered with the occasional sway towards Jackie. Sheer determination and perseverance carried me onward around the nurses' desk. I used the desk as temporary support. Onward bound, I headed towards the toilet. All around me, people were carrying on with normal things. I felt completely outside the normal world. The hazy picture from my weak left eye, the instability of my steps, my trapped mind unable to speak – in my own little world I walked and reached the toilet. I poured my urine into the toilet and, with a push of the toilet handle, I felt triumphant. Completely victorious, I had done it. Walked ten metres without support.

As I walked back to the bed, I could see my parents had just arrived and were watching me. My mother had a concerned look on her face, but I made it back to bed, much to her relief. I collapsed in a heap on the bed. I was mentally and physically fatigued, but supremely proud of my efforts.

I spent a week in Ward A8. During that time, Nick Parkhouse, the crazy plastic surgeon from the QVH, visited me and snipped off the tail of one of the many stitches hanging out of my face. He was pleased with the surgical success of the operation, although concerned, as we all were, about the right-sided weakness of my body.

Arrangements were made for me to return to the QVH for rehabilitation. This time, however, with my life-threatening condition removed, the mode of transport was a normal ambulance. My flying days were over.

On Wednesday, 21 March 1990, I left the Hammersmith Hospital bound for East Grimstead, a whole lot of rehabilitation and who knew what else.

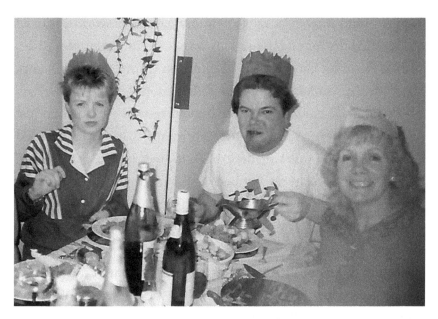

Christmas 1988 – Sharon, me and Mum, before another embolisation.

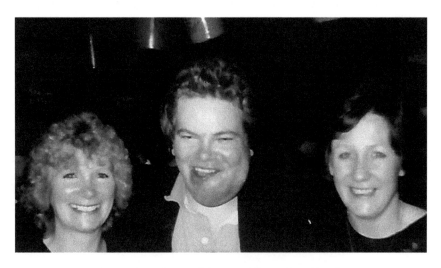

Aunts Rose-Ann and Agnes with me, New Year's
Eve 1989, not long before the big bleed.

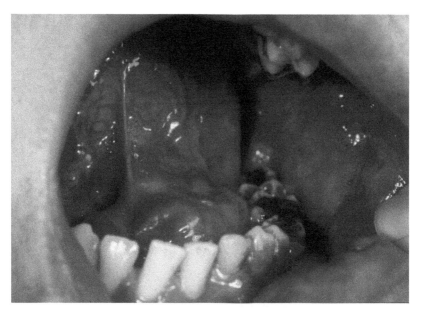

A battle within – arteriovenous malformation invading my
mouth and jaw; teeth displaced by the pressure beneath.

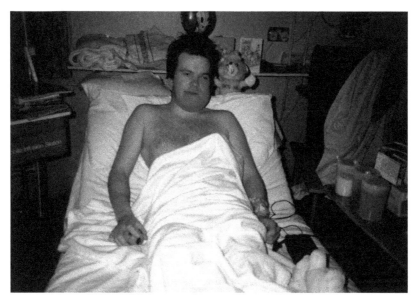

Post major bleed. Decision time.

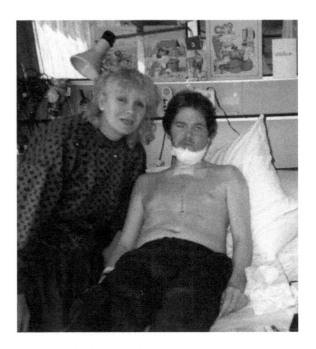

Mum and I celebrate the left eye opening. I can see.

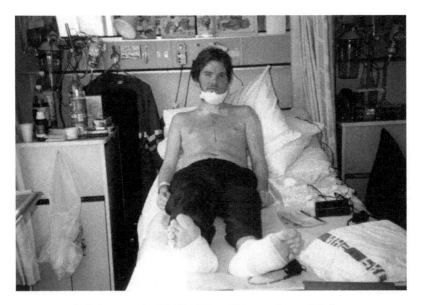

Only in my pain did I find the will to survive and thrive.

PART 3

CHOOSING TO THRIVE

CHAPTER 11

In Recovery

It was a bright sunny day when I arrived back at the QVH. There was a gentle breeze, which struck me because it was the first time I had felt the elements on my body since I had been 'resurrected'.

I was sitting semi-upright on the ambulance trolley, and two ambulance men pushed open the heavy fire doors and pushed me down the long corridor into the main ward. One of the senior nurses on the ward – one I hadn't met during my previous stay – walked towards us at the entrance of the Canadian Wing. With my limited vision, I could barely see her, but I could hear her footsteps. She had a confident walk and a quiet, assertive voice that reassured me.

'Hello, Jerry. My name is Pat. It's nice to meet you. I've heard a lot about you.' This didn't surprise me. I knew the staff would have been talking about my case because of its traumatic nature, especially with Ali having been in the helicopter with me on that dramatic flight to the Hammersmith. No doubt Pat had also heard about how immense the operation had been.

Obviously, I couldn't reply to Pat, but she took the great wad of medical documents the ambulance men gave her, and they carefully moved me from the ambulance trolley and settled me gently into the bed I was to occupy for … who knew how long? It was located diagonally opposite the nurses' office, ideally positioned for observing me. The other advantage was that it was next to a window with a pleasant view out across the gardens, not that I could see it properly at this point.

I settled back in my ward bed, wondering what would come next and what my rehabilitation might look like. Would I ever completely see, speak, eat, drink or walk properly again? What would be my quality of life? I decided right there and then to live for the minute over the coming days, weeks and possibly months, and set small, achievable goals.

The ward was quiet and tranquil that day, which helped settle me in and keep me calm. The many intravenous drips I'd had at the Hammersmith had been removed for the journey to the QVH. The only drip I had at that point was a fluid drip and a cannula (a device used for providing immediate access to the veins).

There was some discussion as to whether I should continue to be fed with a naso-gastric tube. Due to my recent bad experiences of nearly choking to death, I was somewhat loath to. While the naso-gastric tube was out, I attempted a liquidised meal of meat, mash and vegetables, then ice-cream. What a sight I must have been. With every swallow, the food came back up out of the tracheotomy hole in my throat. Sheer frustration drove me to mix the main meal and ice-cream together in a desperate attempt to achieve an acceptable viscosity that would make its way down to my stomach, and this semi-solid mix did seem to work.

It reminded me of staying with Granny in Possilpark when I was finishing my high school exams and could only eat soft food after the first operation. I remember saying to her the mince and tatties (potatoes) she had served were too hot to eat, and she poured milk directly on top of my dinner and said, 'There we go, Jerry. It all goes down the same way anyway.'

I had weighed around eighty-five kilograms before the operation, but I now weighed less than seventy kilograms. This concerned me since my only food intake for some weeks to come would be this delicious cocktail of semi-solids. But I chose to focus on those small, achievable goals. I would simply focus on eating each meal the best I could, trusting that in time, in small incremental steps, I would gain the weight back.

The following day, I had my first bath in weeks. Because I couldn't walk or balance, three nurses helped me into the bath. They were pottering around me, saying things like 'Time for your bath, Jerry' and 'Let's help you along, shall we?' and 'Off we go, Jerry.' It was like a little holiday spa with one of those standalone Victorian clawfoot baths – just me and three nurses … what a dream come true. I lay back and let them bathe me, dry me off and do my hair.

On another occasion soon after I returned to the QVH, my mother – who, along with George, visited almost every day – was brushing my hair, and she noticed a strange mark on my head: three 7s or Ls impressed into my scalp. The surgeons, Brent Tanner and Per Hall, were there, but no one could work out where the 7s had come from. Mum suggested maybe they'd put my head in a clamp during the operation, but Brent Tanner said no, they never clamped people's heads as it would interrupt the blood flow. He said my head had been on a sort of donut pillow to support it. Per Hall shook his head and said he had no idea how it got there but that it was like the branding they do on cattle. Very bizarre. It's visible on my head today and we still don't know how it got there.

By the end of the first week back at the QVH, the extent of the damage to my cranial nerves was fully evident. A weakness of the right leg and arm. An inability to open the right eyelid and speak, eat or drink. The right-hand side of my tongue was also curled up and paralysed, and my right vocal cord was paralysed too. I had developed pressure sores on my ankles and buttocks while at the Hammersmith, so I had bandages and wounds from head to toe. Thankfully, my bed was a waterbed, which helped with the pressure sores.

~

Although I was still in pain and covered in an assortment of wounds, I began my physiotherapy. My physiotherapist was Liz, a tall, thin, grey-haired lady and a highly experienced physio who had worked with many patients who were badly burned. Our first session together, held in the physiotherapy department in a building not far from the Canadian Wing, was simply an assessment of my bodily movements. Liz did not suffer fools gladly, and I was quite happy with that kind of approach. I wanted to work as hard as I could and improve as quickly as I could.

But for the time being, it was about taking tiny, incremental steps. That first session I couldn't walk in a straight line nor very far, perhaps just a few metres. I also felt constantly tired. My hip wound still hadn't healed, and it began to weep after the first physio session, which was a regular occurrence for the next few weeks. But it didn't stop me – I was determined.

I had a stockpile of 'build-up' drinks courtesy of the QVH dietitian. Although I still struggled to swallow anything, I was happy to try any combination of liquid and solids to ensure I ingested some food.

I couldn't speak, so it was time to address this as well. Enter Sue, the speech therapist. Sue had long dark hair and big round spectacles. She was based at another hospital in Tunbridge Wells, but she made special trips to the QVH when required.

Sue was instrumental in my recovery because she showed me how to eat again. She would sit by my bed in the Canadian Wing and teach me to swallow. My epiglottis – the little thing at the top of your throat that lets air into your lungs and then closes so you can swallow and eat – was paralysed as well. So first, she taught me how to place my lips and tongue in the right position for swallowing food. As time went by, she also taught me to move my head down and to the right, which would manually block the entrance to my lungs and keep the entrance to my stomach open to accept food.

As well as learning to eat, I had to learn how to speak again. The sheer frustration of not being able to communicate was massively disheartening for me. Sue explained some lip and tongue exercises, which I carried out daily – simple things like saying the vowels 'A E I O U' over and over, and then doing the same with numbers.

Another exercise involved grunting, which resulted in some amused stares from staff and patients alike in the Canadian Wing. Due to my right vocal cord being paralysed, I grunted to strengthen the left vocal cord. The equipment needed for this exercise was just a chair. The large one next to the bed was perfect. I would sit upright with my arms stretched out on the armrests. I took a deep breath and held the tension, then expelled the air quickly in the form of a grunt. It sounded, and looked, like I had severe constipation, but its effect was remarkable. Immediately after these grunts, I could count to two in my 'old' voice. With continued effort and hard work over a period of weeks, I could soon count to ten without a pause. It would not be long before I could utter a sentence.

~

By the end of my second week, things were slowly improving and it was time to have my facial stitches removed. I looked like a hedgehog, so in some ways I was pleased to hear the stitches were being taken out, although I had no idea what I was in for.

Per Hall came in to assess my face. There were about twenty-five spiky stitch tails visible – thick, nylon gut stitches, generally used for sewing intestines together. He suggested removing several stitches a day, over the next few days, since the removal process would likely be quite painful.

I thought we should get them all out as quickly as possible. More fool me. They ended up doing it over two sessions. It took place in one of the treatment rooms, which I was becoming quite familiar with as I was in there regularly having my dressings changed by Pat, the nurse who had greeted me on arrival. She was assisting Per Hall that day as he selectively cut the stitches.

Each session was a nightmare. My face, having been opened and pulled around in all directions during the operation, was still incredibly tender. They would pinch the skin and pull it right out to get a good angle on the stitch, cut the stitch with scissors and use pliers to pull it out, so my cheek was stretched right out by the time the stitch was released. There was no anaesthetic involved – just normal strength painkillers. It caused acute pain and was quite barbaric, really, but still the best system they had at that time.

I was sweating bullets by the time it was over. When I returned to my bed, I lay there in a trance-like state listening to music, hoping it would drown the painfulness of my throbbing head.

~

On one occasion, as I lay in my bed, I overhead a conversation that touched me deeply. The elderly man in the bed next to me was essentially confined to the hospital. Although he must have been bored beyond belief, he was always cheerful with the staff and my family when they visited. I wished I could communicate with him, but I still couldn't speak properly. Despite the many operations he seemed to have had on his head and face, he maintained his self-respect and dignity. I would think to myself, '*Why do they keep on operating? He's eighty-three!*' I didn't know his medical problem. It just seemed so cruel. Like James, the patient I had met at the Hammersmith who'd had the operation on his liver, this was another situation that brought tears to my eyes. He was so lonely the staff had asked for a voluntary worker to come and speak to him.

One afternoon he was chatting to Di, a nurse, and his tone of voice was low and depressed. He said to her quietly, though I could hear clear enough, 'I wish I could just curl up and die so that I won't be a nuisance to anyone.' My heart sank, and I felt a numbness come over me. Although he was eighty-three years old, he had no one – no family, no friends – to visit him or care for him. I thought of when he was born – he'd been someone's little boy. I imagined the happiness he must have brought into his parents' life. Now to see him with only half a face undergoing even more operations, I felt so sad for him. He died a few months later. Life can be so cruel sometimes. When you are young, it's easier to find hope for the future. For our aged folk, there has to be a better way, especially when they are so isolated and in pain.

～

By the end of my second week in the Canadian Wing, my communication had improved. I still had the dressing on my jaw and tracheotomy site. My barely audible voice was understandable if I paused after each faintly heard word. I was impressed with myself, although normal conversation was a non-starter. On a Sunday afternoon, my parents wheeled me outside to the grassy area just outside the ward. To feel the flow of air over my body was immensely refreshing and that afternoon I spent a few hours soaking up the sunrays. Two friends, Tom Richardson and Vic Young, arrived while I was still sitting outside, and they were surprised to see me up and about. When they had last visited at the Hammersmith, I'd been in a vegetative state.

Later that evening, while speaking to a nurse, I noticed my voice wasn't as strong as it had been – in fact, alarmingly, it seemed to be disappearing. Soon, I couldn't get any sound out. Even though my jaw and lips were moving in an effort to speak, not even a whisper could be heard. I was devastated. The ear, nose and throat consultant suggested we wait six months to see if any improvement was evident, and, if not, there was the possibility of injecting my paralysed right vocal chord with Teflon (more typically used on non-stick frying pans), which would improve my ability to speak. I did not like the sound of that. Surely if my voice had returned once, it would again?

The following day I began to develop chest pain, which soon intensified and became quite alarming. The pain was immobilising. The doctors thought it was a chest infection, possibly pneumonia – certainly not ideal after major surgery and having my chest opened up for a heart-lung bypass. They suggested perhaps being out in the grounds on Sunday afternoon had exposed me to the germs and infections present outside.

At the same time, I had an infection on my chest due to the hair follicles growing on my chest scar. This resulted in my chest being painted with Betadine, an iodine-based solution used as skin preparation in theatres before surgery.

For the next week, I was bed bound except for visits to the dressing room. With this crippling pain, I honestly thought I was going downhill rapidly. I was prescribed antibiotics along with the old remedy of a bowl of hot water with a menthol inhaler, which helped with breathing, and a week later I was back on course for a steady recovery. It certainly explained why my voice had disappeared and I was grateful to find that, as I recovered, so did my voice.

~

It was always a good day when I received a postcard from Steve Rigg. His cards would bring shouts of 'outrageous', 'shocking' and 'should be banned' from the nursing staff. 'How could the postal service handle them?' they asked. It's not that they were pornographic – just tasteful black-and-white postcards of gorgeous, pouting, partially clad females. Well, okay, some of them were topless ... but they brought a smile to my face and I suppose that's the main thing. Over time a collection started to grow in the ward. I liked to think some of the other patients loved it as much as I did, because they started asking when the next one would arrive. And I enjoyed sharing them around.

I had acquired some wheels in the form of a wheelchair. Unfortunately, I couldn't 'do it up' with stickers and the pornographic postcards because it was shared between a number of patients. I didn't have the strength to wheel myself around, so a nurse or another patient would take me for a 'wheel about'.

My first visit to the TV room gave me a real shock. The nurse had kindly put the brakes on and was about to leave me. I looked down at my thighs and I saw a hand resting on my right thigh for what seemed a long time. I thought, '*Why is her hand there and why hasn't she removed it?*' I turned to my right to see what she was up to. She was almost out the door. '*Well, whose hand was it then?*' I couldn't work it out. I followed the hand up to the shoulder – then realised it was *my* hand. I was shocked. I couldn't believe it was my hand. In a frightful state, I called out for a nurse in my usual inarticulate and uncoordinated voice to explain what I was experiencing. Pat and a doctor came in to see me. The doctor suggested that, given all my brain had been through, its signals and muscular movements were still not fully operational. It was an eye-opener for me, but, in the end, I saw it as a positive thing – just another step on my journey towards healing.

~

Another significant milestone, achieved at the end of my third week at the QVH, was the closing up of my tracheotomy hole. Then five weeks post-operation, it was time for the big reveal. Pat was going to be removing the dressing as the wound had healed. She called in anyone who was around to come and see, and we had a mini-celebration in the dressing room. I was unimpressed with the rejoicing, however. After all, I still couldn't speak properly and there was a lot of necrotic tissue on my jaw. Dressings were applied daily on those areas to encourage the tissues to gradually fall off. The necrotic tissue was a result of too much STD (the gluing agent they use for varicose veins) that was used on my face during the operation, hence the good skin had also been eaten away.

The stench of the necrotic tissue was like something long dead as if the body was decomposing while still alive. That was likely the cause of the high temperatures and heavy sweats I was having. It was time for the remaining hard necrotic tissue to be removed. Brent Tanner started cutting away the skin with a pair of surgical scissors under no anaesthetic. Lying on the bed in the dressing room of the Canadian Wing, Tanner's senior registrar held my head still while Pat passed the surgical instruments. Tanner pulled and cut the skin from my jaw while my whole body underwent some sort of physical convulsive shock wave.

It was like rust repair work on a car. To get rid of the rust, you have to go right down to the metal base. You can't leave any of the rust there because it will just return. So you almost have to take a layer of steel off to get rid of the rust. It was the same with my face. They had to cut right down near the bone to remove the dead tissue. My eyes were watering as he cut. I was so tensed up that water flowed out of my eyes. I was in so much pain. I couldn't breathe I was so tense. *Snip, snip, snip.* Just when I thought my physical pain was on the decrease, it shot up rapidly yet again. *'When would it all be over?'*

CHAPTER 12

Getting to Know Pat

Pat had become an important part of my recovery. She was the person who changed all my surgical dressings – on my chest, neck, face and even the pressure sores on my ankles and bum! So for a couple of hours a day, I was closeted in this little dressing room area with her. She would remove all the old dressings, clean my wounds and then do fresh dressings.

I couldn't speak to her at first – nor see her properly. Then, as the tracheotomy healed, I began to speak a little. My speech was very slurred, very stop-start, but at least I could express myself ever so slightly. I could only manage one word at a time and had to take a big breath of air to force the words out because of the paralysis of the vocal cord. It was an awful lot of effort. When I started to speak again, at first there was no accent at all. It was all very hoarse, almost a whisper. In time, as my speech improved, Pat said to me one day, 'You've got a Scottish accent!'

She hadn't realised I was Scottish and my accent seemed to get a good reception from her, so I milked it for all it was worth. I tried rolling my 'r's in that Scottish way, which seemed to make her smile. So I tried making up some ridiculous phrases with as many 'r's in them as possible, like: 'Dirty turtles eating burgers in murky water.' Pat would smile briefly and then immediately carry on with changing my dressings. Always the consummate professional. She was so efficient that it was difficult to get much out of her. She was one of the youngest ward sisters, so she must have felt that professional responsibility of being in charge of the whole ward at such a young age.

I started thinking, '*What the hell can I do to make this woman laugh?*' She was very polite, but trying to crack a joke or engage in some banter was redundant. You couldn't tell if she liked you or disliked you. And I liked her. From the start, I liked her. Even before I could see her. I just liked her presence.

She couldn't stick anything on my face to hold the dressings on and that's why I ended up with a big bow around my head, holding everything together. It was a bandage that went under my chin and tied like a bow on top of my head. She and the other nurses played around with different bow styles. Then I had to walk around the ward like that and we all had a bit of a laugh.

Around that time, one of my university colleagues, Richard Whitehead, came to visit me and Pat was on the ward that day. As she walked past, I turned to Richard and said, 'I'm going to marry that woman.' I don't know why. I can't explain it. Maybe you can't help who you fall in love with. There is no scientific equation for love. It is not something that follows a recipe or that you can manufacture.

Mind you, I had no idea how I was going to make it happen. I wasn't exactly a catch in my situation. I'd been near to death on many occasions and, if I did survive, I had an uncertain future. But I wasn't about to let that get in the way of what I wanted.

Perhaps it gave me even more incentive to throw myself into my physiotherapy training. The pressure sores on my ankles were healing but, to an extent, the physio work conflicted with the healing process. Because of all the dressings, stitches and scars, when you're stretching things and moving your body around during physio, it can counter the healing process by pulling at the stitches. But then if you don't do any exercises, you get weaker and weaker, so it was a conundrum. The situation had to be carefully monitored, which both Liz and I did. For example, there was a device with a little ball inside that you'd blow into – like if you get stopped by a booze bus and you have to blow into a tube. The aim was to push the ball out using your breath. But it would break down the scar tissue on my chest, so that was a problem. I wanted to get strong quickly, but I also didn't want to mess with the healing process.

In the early stages, my physio consisted of stretching exercises and learning to walk up and down some steps. Although I could walk a short distance, I was sluggish, with my head hanging over and an ungainly gait. The stretching exercises improved this. In the physiotherapy department, there were these training steps I would climb, holding Liz's hand, and that's how I learned to walk up and down stairs all over again.

The workout increased to twice daily as I improved. The morning session consisted of balance and coordination exercises with Liz. For the balance exercises, I would stand on a gym bench and Liz would run around the bench, throwing rings and balls for me to turn around and catch. The afternoon session involved some light weights for building up my general strength. Although the strength of my left hand was okay, I could only manage a half-kilo weight in my right hand.

Before the operation, I had played soccer for leisure with work colleagues and friends. Now just kicking a light football to Liz was frustrating, let alone any effort to dribble a football around three cones. I stumbled again and again in my uncoordinated way. But eventually, with perseverance and single-mindedness, the results became evident, which only served to increase my determination. I became a man obsessed with the sole aim of being 'normal'.

Liz created a miniature obstacle course for me, comprising small objects that might be a trip hazard. This was an excellent test as Liz would time my runs. The obstacle course involved crawling, running, jumping and balancing, and I was improving my time on each go. Liz, with a stopwatch in hand, would shout and cajole me into faster and faster times. I left the physio department in a state of physio-shock, in pain and exhausted, but always with a tremendous feeling of achievement and satisfaction. I would continue with the physio until I couldn't take it anymore. On more than one occasion, after pushing too hard, I was actually physically sick. This didn't concern me; it just meant I was working hard and would soon see even better results.

The Canadian Wing was a long Nightingale ward with patio-type doors that opened up onto the grounds. Part of the recovery for the pilots back in Archibald McIndoe's day had involved them being able to go outside, sit on the grass and take in the summer sunshine. So I would go out there and do extra physio. I'd take a soccer ball with me and pass it around my waist while walking to increase dexterity and coordination, or throw the ball in the air and try to catch it. Trying to run was quite funny, as the right-hand side of my body would lag behind the left. I must have looked like one of those slinky springs we used in physics class at school.

The hospital grounds also played host to my golfing abilities. I asked my parents to bring me a putter, and I dug some small holes in the ground. The flags were made from cut bin liners stuck onto branches on nearby trees. Most afternoons you'd find me putting a golf ball and soaking up the sunrays.

~

In parallel with my physical progress, my right eye was showing signs of opening. Over the period of a week, it began to open. A truly miraculous event if ever there was one. I had already had my left eye tested for a pair of spectacles to improve the vision of the left eye, since I'd almost resigned myself to the fact that I would only have one eye. The right eye gradually opened up completely, although full vision had not returned. At first, I had double vision, which was rather unnerving as I would continually bump into chairs and doors. Secondly, I had limited movement of the pupil.

After a few days off, Pat returned on a late shift, and she was walking around saying hello to everybody. She stopped and turned around when she saw me and said, 'Your eyes are open!' I just smiled – I could see her much better. My eyesight was a little blurry still, but it was lovely to get a proper look at her.

I was attracted to her large, beautiful eyes. Some people find other body parts attractive (and don't get me wrong, other physical attributes are indeed appealing), and I guess we are all different, but I'm attracted to eyes. Eyes never really change during your lifetime; other body parts change in shape and size, but eyes stay the same. Eyes don't lie; they are honest. No matter what someone tells you, what they genuinely feel can be seen in the first few milliseconds in their eyes. I also see (no pun intended) the eyes as a gateway to the soul. If you look behind a person's eyes, you will see them for who they really are and establish if they are a good human. Pat was a good human. I could see it in her eyes and feel it in her touch as she changed my dressings.

The fear of not being able to see again had been the worst feeling. I thought I could probably live with being disabled or not being able to move my arm or leg, but there's something about sight, the ability to see, that is so important. It's the key way we make sense of the world, how we envision the world we live in and how we consolidate what we take in through our other senses. Maybe if you were born blind, you could develop your other senses, but to lose your sight as an adult must be so hard. Especially when there's nothing you can do about it – you can't work on your sight returning the way you can work on your body with physiotherapy. It's a binary thing – either on or off, no in-between. I was so relieved and grateful when my sight returned. It actually made everything else easier thereafter – the physio, the whole recovery. It was such a motivation to continue getting better and better.

~

Part of the therapy the QVH provided was encouragement to get out in public even if you were bandaged up and scarred. There was a pub nearby known as the Guinea Pig. It had been there since Archibald McIndoe's days when they started the Guinea Pig drinking club for the pilots and aviators he operated on, encouraging them to go out into the community and engage with the locals, despite their facial deformities. I used to go there for a drink with some of the other patients sometimes. One night Pat was there with some of the other nurses and that's when I decided

I would have to do something about my interest in her. I needed to come up with a plan and make my move ... I just wasn't sure what that move might be.

~

In the meantime, life in the QVH continued, along with my recovery. Towards the end of my stay, a Greek woman with an AVM came into the hospital. Brent Tanner was getting a reputation following the operation he did on me, and patients were being referred to him. The woman's daughter was in her early twenties with long dark hair and attractive features. She'd come into the Canadian Wing and ask Pat where I was.

Pat would direct her out to the gardens or wherever and we'd go for a walk. I found out later Pat thought I had a 'thing' going on with the Greek goddess. But the truth was, she wanted to find out as much as she could about AVMs for her mother's sake. Her mum's AVM was in her throat. If it bled, she could choke to death, so the young woman was just trying to glean as much information as possible to help her mother.

She asked me questions about my AVM and the treatment, and I told her about embolisation, which I figured was a technique that could be used for her mother, since I couldn't see how surgery would work – how do you get access to inside somebody's throat and tie off those vessels? When I think about that poor woman, I realise how lucky I actually was that mine was at least operable – even though the operation nearly killed me.

~

Towards the end of my time at the QVH, a bunch of actors showed up one day. They were making a TV series set at the hospital called *A Perfect Hero*, and all the actors who were playing pilots and aviators from the Second World War were very handsome. One of them was Nigel Havers, who'd been in *Chariots of Fire*.

The series showed how burn victims were treated and how they had to recuperate. Havers played a character called Fleming, who was once an extremely handsome young man who had no problem dating women. With his face deformed by burns and the subsequent plastic surgery, his life became rather more traumatic. Now that was something I related to.

Some of the actors had crutches and bandages, and I was there hanging around trying to get in on it because I figured I was the genuine article. I didn't even need makeup or anything. I remember thinking, '*Well, look, you've got the real thing here … why don't you ask me to participate?*'

But it wasn't to be. My famous actor dreams were thwarted before they'd even begun.

~

As further preparation for returning to normal life out of hospital, I was allowed weekend leave while I built up my physical strength. My parents, who had visited me nearly every day at the QVH, were relieved I could come home to Stanmore Park and they didn't have to travel to East Grinstead for the weekends anymore.

One weekend I even managed a trip to Rugby. Richard Drabble was having a party and George drove me up on the Saturday. Things were really getting back to normal – I could even dance. There was no stopping me when 'Love Shack' by the B-52s came on. My speech was still husky and with no power, and I still had a bandage on my face, albeit much smaller. I was grateful I no longer had to wear the bow on my head, though I'm sure my friends would've found it highly amusing. It was a mad weekend, to be honest. Richard had invited everybody that I worked with and we all got a bit raucous. I remember jumping on somebody's back at one point, dancing and partying. Many people stayed over – they all just crashed where they were. Bodies piled up everywhere: five or six people in a bed, on settees, on floors.

But the best bit about it all was just getting to see and speak to my friends again and being able to feel like a normal twenty-something person. It was indeed a special moment in my recovery.

CHAPTER 13

Matters of the Heart

The more my health improved and the more I got to know her, the more I thought about asking Pat out, but I still didn't know how to broach the subject.

During one of our sessions when she was changing my dressings, as a way of testing the waters, I propositioned her (no, not marriage). My friend, Steve Cook, who had moved to New York for work, had asked me to fly over for a visit once I'd left the hospital. So I said to Pat, 'I've been invited to the States to visit a friend who recently moved there. Would you like to come with me?' I was just sounding her out, really, to see what she would say, so I said it in a jokey way – not too serious, but sort of semi-serious…

The problem was, she thought I was fully joking. Just another patient trying to chat her up. So that ploy went nowhere, though perhaps it's also when she started to cotton on that I liked her.

My next attempt was to ask her out for a drink, to which she agreed, but then she showed up with two other nurses: Liz, her best friend who also looked after me in the Russell Davies Unit – the one who squeezed my zits – and Steve. We went to the White Horse Inn and I suppose I was 'doing the groundwork' for what I hoped would follow. But as we left the pub, I bottled out. I wanted to tell her how I felt, but I just didn't. I blew it. When I returned to the ward in the wee small hours of the morning, I was not happy with myself.

Then I heard there was a party coming up for Greg, the charge nurse, who was leaving to go to another hospital. This would be an excellent opportunity to approach her, I thought. But yet again, there didn't seem to be an opportunity to make a move.

I was getting desperate. I would be leaving the hospital in the next week or so, and I wanted to let her know how I felt before I did. I racked my brain for a game plan, and I came up with the idea of hosting a leaving barbecue. Instead of buying the nursing staff chocolates and cards for looking after me, I'd invite them all to a barbecue. Genius! I asked various people to nip out to the shops and purchase the sausages and drinks at my expense. The scene was set. The barbecue was to be held in the gardens behind the nursing accommodation. To add a bit of fun, I organised some party games: wheelbarrow races, egg and spoon, and a three-legged rugby match using a football.

The nursing staff, along with the maxillofacial and plastic surgeons, all eagerly joined in the fun and frivolity. Dr Gately, the duty plastic surgeon on that night, even joined in on the games in his blue surgical scrubs.

As things quietened down and it started to get dark and a little chilly, most partygoers moved inside to the nurses' quarters to dance. Pat was still sitting outside with a few others, and I just thought, '*Carpe diem, Jerry … it's now or never – go for it!*'

While the others were talking among themselves, I asked her quietly if we could have a little chat and she agreed. So far so good. I led her around the corner and up a little hill to a bench seat outside the burns unit.

I could tell she was cold, wearing only a t-shirt and shorts, and

I didn't want the poor girl to suffer, so I just came out with it: 'I'd like to see you when I leave the hospital,' I said. 'I like you and want to get to know you more...' No reading between the lines. I knew how fragile life could be and how time was a precious commodity. To my surprise and sheer delight, she didn't say no. In fact, she seemed quite receptive to the idea.

But then she threw a spanner in the works. 'There's something I need to tell you though, Jerry...'

'What?' I said, thinking, '*Oh no, things were going so well.*' What could it be?

'It's just ... there's another man in my life...'

'*What the hell?*' I thought, my heart sinking...

'He's only about three foot tall though...'

Upon further explanation, it turned out the three-foot-tall 'man' was in fact her son, a five-year-old named Stephen, and, clearly, she was wondering if that would be an issue.

Without hesitation, I said, 'It's not a problem, Pat. The way I see it, if you truly care for someone, it doesn't matter how many kids they've got. Don't worry about it ... let's just see what the future brings.'

Pat smiled, visibly relaxing. 'Jerry Morrissey – you're a good man,' she said, and with that we leaned in and hugged and kissed for the first time.

I couldn't believe it was all working out just the way I'd hoped. But the night was getting colder, and I wanted to spend more time with her, so I took off back down the hill at a slow and steady trot to the ward to grab some jumpers. I wanted her to feel warm and comfortable as we snuggled under the starry sky.

When I got back, I asked her if she wanted a drink, and she thought perhaps I'd grabbed an orange juice from my bedside locker. I walked over to the bushes and pulled out a bottle of chilled sparkling wine, accompanied by two wine glasses wrapped in a tea towel. A few hours earlier, I'd stashed the bottle in the bushes along with a big ice-filled water jug from the ward, in anticipation of a romantic night. We chatted about each other's lives as we drank the wine. There was something about this woman – even though I hardly knew her – that made me feel so comfortable. It just felt so *right* being with her.

We didn't tell anyone about our budding romance, as Pat didn't want her professional reputation to be put at risk, and forming a relationship with a patient could potentially be frowned upon. Later that week, when I left the hospital, we could 'go public'.

～

For my last night at the QVH, I had arranged a dinner date with Pat at the Monsoon Restaurant, a local Indian place. I changed my pyjamas for some clothes my parents had brought in specially – a blue blazer, red and grey striped shirt, chinos and brogues, which clicked as I strode along the hard floors of the Canadian Wing, giving me an air of authority, which I enjoyed. Pat and I snuck out of the hospital – me still with a big dressing on my face. As we entered the restaurant, I could tell people were staring, but I didn't care.

After perusing the menu for a few minutes, I asked Pat what she wanted to order.

'I can't make up my mind what to have for starters or main,' she said, 'but I know what I want for dessert.'

'Okay,' I said, 'let's have our meal backwards then.' Pat chuckled dubiously, no doubt thinking I wasn't being serious.

When the waiter arrived, I asked for two Irish coffees and ordered a dessert each. 'What about your starter and main course, sir?' said the waiter.

'We'd like to have the meal backwards actually, starting with coffee, then dessert, main course and starters.'

'Don't you like our main dishes, sir?'

'Yes, but we would like to eat backwards tonight,' I said, decisively.

He nodded his head. 'Very good, sir.' Then I heard him speaking to one of his colleagues at the bar, probably telling him they had a couple of weirdos in the restaurant. With the bandage on my face, my scars and wounds still visible, and my voice low and husky, he probably thought I wasn't the 'full shilling'. Then there was the fact that I had to move my head around at strange angles to swallow, as Sue, the speech therapist, had shown me. I must have looked quite the sight to the other customers and staff. But again, I didn't care – I was just focused on Pat and the two of us having a good time.

After dinner, we walked around the hospital grounds, stopping to hug each other in a passionate embrace and kiss, then I walked her home since she lived just around the corner from the hospital with her parents and son. It was late when I got back to the ward. A senior nurse manager who didn't know me thought I was a doctor as I walked into the Canadian Wing – must've been the blue blazer and the click of the shoes. That night I lay awake thinking about Pat and the future we would have together, and wondering how life would be when I left the hospital the very next day.

～

On Friday, 18 May 1990, I was discharged from the QVH as an in-patient. Pat was working on the early shift and helped me pack all my belongings into my parents' car that afternoon. We said goodbye although it wouldn't be long before we saw each other again, as we had planned for me to meet her parents and five-year-old son, Stephen.

My plan of action was to stay with my parents at RAF Stanmore Park, a couple of hours' drive up the road from Pat. I would take a few weeks to hang out and relax before I went back up to Warwickshire, to Rugby, and back to work, though I wasn't sure when that would happen. After all, my job involved managing major projects and a considerable number of meetings and telephone calls, so I needed to have my voice in proper working order.

Therefore, the most important aspect of rehabilitation was regaining my voice. Still hoarse, husky and barely audible, it was improving but would take quite some time to fully recover. My plan was also to increase the physio exercises to get back to normal strength. In Stanmore Park, my bedroom was on the first floor, so just getting up and down the stairs was like physio, and I planned to climb them over and over.

For the next couple of months, I commuted from my parents' house to East Grinstead to visit Pat and have regular check-ups with the maxillofacial and plastic surgeons.

The first time I met Stephen, I could see just how much he looked like Pat with those characteristically large eyes. Apparently, he'd been very excited about meeting me and our planned day out. He was very polite and well-mannered, and acted more like a middle-aged man than a kid. With Pat working full-time, other than school, he spent most of his time with his grandparents, Rosemary and Norman.

Our first day out as a threesome was fun. We went to a nearby park for a picnic and to play some games, which broke the ice. One particularly frustrating moment for me, though, was when I tried to lift Stephen over the fence to the picnic area, and my right side, still weak from the stroke, gave way. I'd been overly ambitious thinking I could bear his weight, and I just wasn't ready for that. It seemed I still had plenty of work to do to get my strength back.

All was progressing well except for my relationship with Pat's parents, who did not seem that keen on me. My easy-going, extroverted style conflicted with their narrow-minded Victorian attitudes. I suppose I came across as not a very serious person. They seemed to think I was a fly-by-night character only interested in 'one thing' with Pat. I must have seemed like a tornado coming into this straight-laced family: the picnics, the days out, the new ideas of what to do. It seemed like it was just too much for her parents to take on board, especially her mother.

I still hadn't taken that trip to New York to stay with Steve Cook. When I mentioned it again to Pat, this time she said 'yes' to coming with me. We started planning – it would be the holiday of a lifetime. We would stay with Steve, who had a high-flying advertising job, and his girlfriend, Anita, and live it up in the Big Apple for a couple of weeks.

But Pat's parents did not approve, and they made it a major guilt-trip operation. How could Pat possibly leave her five-year-old son for two weeks? It was irresponsible … outrageous. What sort of a mother would do that?

When that didn't work – I saw right through what they were doing – they made it difficult in other areas. Pat didn't have a passport and since she had been born in Canada, she needed to show her parents' marriage certificate to obtain one. I'd bought the plane tickets and everything was organised apart from a trip to the passport office. But Pat's parents refused to give her their marriage certificate.

Pat was distraught. I met her at a coffee shop in East Grinstead and she was crying. I didn't know at this point what was going on. I was assuming she and I would soon be off to London to organise a passport.

Pat began pouring her heart out about her parents and their attitude. I couldn't believe how petty they were being. Pat had met someone who not only cared for her but was willing to take on the responsibility of her five-year-old son. She hadn't been on a holiday for years, ever since Stephen had been born. In fact, she'd only been on one holiday in her entire twenty-six years on Earth – a mini break to Wales. All she did was work at that hospital and look after Stephen and her parents. I was thinking, '*For God's sake, give the girl a break – she really needs it.*' It wasn't as if she was leaving… just getting on a flight and having a little holiday.

We left the coffee shop and went to the local park and sat on a park bench without saying much. I held her hand and just let her know I was there for her. She was in such a state and I was pondering the situation – trying to get my head around the mentality of her parents. I was also weighing up my options. I could give them what they wanted and say my goodbyes, never to be seen again (not really an option, but it was always part of my thinking to weigh up all the possible scenarios before deciding on the best course of action). Or I could go back to her parents' house and confront them. This seemed like the only viable alternative, so I jumped up and said, 'Let's go!'

'Where?' said Pat.

'We're going back to your parents' house to sort this out.'

Her eyes widened, anticipating the reaction of her parents, but she agreed.

On entering the house, I encountered her mother.

'Where's Norman?' I said.

'He's in the garden,' she said, and I told her I thought we should all sit down and have a talk.

I explained how their attitude was affecting Pat and tried to get them to see reason. But it was too emotional and personal for them and they didn't want to discuss it. They couldn't see I genuinely cared for their daughter and wanted to take care of her and Stephen. I was starting to suspect they just didn't want Pat and Stephen to leave, and I was a threat because I was taking them away. I couldn't understand how they could see it that way – surely they could look at it as gaining a son-in-law?

But they wouldn't listen, and I could see how upset Pat was getting. It seemed there was no way forward that we could forge together, so I let them know exactly where things stood.

'I don't give a shit about what you or anyone else thinks or does – the only thing I'm concerned about is me, Pat and Stephen,' I said.

After everything I had been through, nearly losing my life, intense physical and emotional pain, the stroke and months of rehabilitation, I had finally found happiness with Pat, and she had found happiness with me. And now her parents seemed intent on destroying it.

CHAPTER 14

Love in the Face of Adversity

About six months after I left the hospital, I started to think about proposing to Pat. I was back at work in Rugby, I'd been to New York to stay with Steve Cook – without Pat unfortunately – and my voice had kept on improving, as had my strength and agility.

I asked one of Pat's friends, a nurse called Jo Vaughan, to invite Pat out for a meal at the White Horse. My plan was to turn up unannounced and ask Pat to marry me.

However, Pat was feeling a bit off-colour on the day, so Jo contacted me to say she wasn't going to be there after all. (Unbeknown to me at the time, Pat had found out she'd had an abnormal pap smear result and would have to get treatment.) I asked Jo to let her in on part of the secret to entice her there, and Pat eventually agreed to come out that night knowing I wanted to surprise her with my visit. She just didn't know why…

I called the owner of the White Horse to fill him in on my plans, just to ensure that everything ran smoothly. Pat and I were regulars since it was quite close to Pat's parents' place and we would often drop in for a meal when I was visiting on the weekend.

I'd bought a blue topaz engagement ring, which wasn't expensive, since I didn't earn a lot of money in those days as a graduate trainee, but it was pretty and I thought Pat would like it.

I was nervous when I arrived at the White Horse – and all day before that too. What if she said no? You just never really knew what was going on in someone else's head. From my point of view, she was the person I wanted to spend the rest of my life with, so I was determined to ask her, and I was *fairly* confident she would say 'yes'. I saw the owner out of the corner of my eye as I walked in, and he nodded at me, a grin on his face.

I sat down at the table the owner had booked for us and waited for Pat to arrive. Tapping my foot in anticipation, I looked out across the glass floor, which was actually a giant aquarium, filled with water. As I gazed at the koi carp fish swimming around underfoot, I saw the door open and in she walked.

She was subdued at first, not surprising considering the news she'd had that day. But once we ordered some food and chatted about her health and the treatment she would need, we both started to relax. By the time dessert had arrived, it felt like the right time, so I pulled out the ring and opened the box. Pat was looking at me wide-eyed with a half-smile on her face as I showed her the contents.

'Will you marry me, Pat?' I said, no mucking around.

She smiled at me fully then, but there was a long pause… '*Don't leave me hanging here*,' I thought. I felt like I was going to have a heart attack or my heart was going to pump right out of my chest and all those stitches would break. Lord knows we didn't need to call an ambulance that night.

'Yes!' she said, eventually. Apparently, she'd had no idea I was going to propose.

The owner and a few of the service staff had been keeping a close eye on me, waiting for the proposal. When they saw the ring going onto Pat's finger, they raced over with a bottle of champagne and popped the cork.

I was ecstatic – she'd said yes and we were going to get married!

~

But not everyone was as happy as we were. When Pat told her parents, her mother, Rosemary, said, 'Why do you want to marry *him*? Have you considered he might die in the next couple of years? What has he got to offer you?'

But as time went on, they seemed to adjust to the idea and offered to help financially. Pat's dad, Norman, said he would give us a five per cent deposit on a house or they would pay for the wedding. Being practical, I thought we should take the deposit money, but Pat wanted a church wedding. So in the end, her parents made all the bookings on our behalf, much to Pat's frustration as her mother barely consulted her when making decisions about our big day.

One Sunday morning, we were at their house discussing the wedding over a cup of tea. By this stage, Pat and Stephen had moved to Rugby to live with me in anticipation of the upcoming nuptials. Again, Rosemary and Norman had expressed their disapproval, but they were starting to realise we were committed and this wedding would be going ahead.

Rosemary pulled out a brochure and showed us the car she had booked for the big day, without consulting Pat or me.

'But I really like the other car,' said Pat, 'and it's cheaper too.'

'Oh, well, never mind,' said Rosemary. 'We've ordered it now, and we're the ones paying for it.'

That was the end of every conversation on the subject: 'We're the ones paying for it.' Next we moved on to talk about the guest list. Rosemary wasn't happy that I had so many family members and friends on the list, and she wanted to invite the neighbours and some other friends Pat and I didn't even know. Pat had met my extended family. She thought they were really welcoming, lovely people and she wanted them to come. The neighbours had no meaning for her at all, and she told her mother that. It didn't go down well; her mother probably thought I was masterminding the whole thing and manipulating Pat.

Tempers, which had been pushed down for the sake of being polite, were simmering away madly underneath – and then things just blew up.

'That's it, I've had enough,' shouted Rosemary. 'I'm going to cancel the wedding. And you can both get out of my house right now!'

She'd been spoiling for an argument because she felt I was taking Pat and Stephen away. The same thing had happened with her son. When he'd announced he was getting engaged, Pat's parents didn't approve nor did they go to his wedding. Pat was meant to be one of the bridesmaids and that got pulled as well. It was history repeating itself.

Okay, well, if they wanted us to leave, leave we would. Pat ran upstairs to pack her wedding dress. Then as we went out to the car to load up, Rosemary flung Pat's wedding shoes out the front door at us and said, 'You better take these with you.' She followed that up with, 'But you can leave Stephen here with me.'

'He's not your child. He's mine,' said Pat, with a steely look in her eye as she hustled Stephen into the car.

Rosemary turned to me and shouted, 'None of Pat's friends like you anyway. You're egotistical!'

I couldn't help myself. I turned back around and said, 'You forgot to add, "You're an egotistical fat git!"'

It was becoming blatantly clear what the whole thing was about: she wanted to keep Stephen and raise him as her own. And whether she had anything more to do with us or not was purely academic. She didn't want to be left alone with Norman. It wasn't a happy marriage, and Pat and Stephen's presence in the home was a buffer. She had tried many times to leave when Pat was younger, but by this point she had just resigned herself to the situation.

We were shellshocked and not sure what to do next. We drove around East Grinstead, looking for a cafe where we could sit down and process what had just happened. The Happy Eater was open, so we went in for a coffee.

Pat was distraught and in tears. We speculated whether it had been her parents' plan all along … to lead us into a false sense of security by offering financial support and then withdrawing and cancelling everything so the wedding could not go ahead.

Then we discussed whether we should just go back to Rugby. I suggested we should see the vicar first to tell him the wedding was off. Since it was Sunday morning, Father Richard Arrandale was at St Swithun's Church, where we were going to get married. He was about to take the ten o'clock church service when we arrived.

'Hi, Father,' I said. 'We're here because we just wanted to let you know the wedding's off,' I said, my arm around Pat, who was still in tears.

Father Richard looked a little taken aback at this and said, 'Look, hang on … here's my house keys. Go back to my house. This is the address. Wait there and when I'm finished with the church service, I'll come and have a chat.'

We'd met Father Richard a few times over the last few months to talk about things and prepare for marriage, so we'd got to know each other a little and he seemed like a good man. We went up to his house and waited. When he returned an hour or two later, he pulled out a pen and notebook and sat with his head on one side, listening to what we had to say.

When we had finished telling him the story, he said, 'If there's one wedding that must happen, it's this wedding. The wedding must go on.'

'But we can't afford it,' I said. 'Pat's parents were paying for everything.'

They had booked the reception at East Court Mansion, a big old house, like a country estate, within walking distance of Pat's house. They'd also organised a photographer, caterers, vehicles and so on.

'Don't worry about that,' he said. 'We'll get everything sorted. The church fees – we'll waive those for starters. And you don't need to worry about flowers; there's a wedding booked just before yours. The church will be full of flowers anyway, so we can just use those. You can stay here the night before the wedding, and, Jerry, your family can join you here on the day to get ready if they wish. You let me know what hymns you want and I'll tell the organist.'

One by one, he listed everything we needed to take care of and came up with a solution. We couldn't believe how kind he was being. He even offered us a place to stay for the next six weeks if we needed it, which we thanked him for, but we had the house in Rugby to return to.

By the time we left, thanks to the true Christian values Father Richard had shown us, we were confident the wedding would go ahead.

Once we got back to Rugby and adjusted to the new plans, I asked Steve Rigg, my best man, to take the wedding photos. Steve was an amateur photographer, and he was more than happy to handle the photography.

Father Richard had said we could use the church garden for the reception if we wanted to. However, when we spoke to the people at East Court Mansion, it turned out Pat's parents had paid a non-refundable deposit. We couldn't afford to make up the difference for an evening reception, so we negotiated the cheapest deal we could get for a finger buffet. And to reduce the cost further, we agreed to clean all the dishes and glasses afterwards.

Steve Cook, who was getting paid very well in his advertising job in New York, stepped in and told us to pick anywhere in the world we wanted to go and he'd pay for our honeymoon as a wedding gift. Pat was overwhelmed by this level of generosity – as was I, to be honest. What great friends we had! We pondered what to book and decided on Vienna, since neither of us had been there before, and we were interested in the history and architecture. Plus, it was in Europe, so it wouldn't be that expensive.

The plans were all taken care of – it was going to be a great wedding.

~

But before the wedding could take place, there were a few more dramas to contend with. Pat and Stephen had quickly adjusted to life in Rugby, and Pat was doing some agency work at St Cross, the general hospital in Rugby where I'd ended up with the massive bleed prior to the operation. Stephen was going to the local Rokeby Primary School (the ancient name for Rugby) and had quickly integrated and made friends.

One day, I was standing at the top of the stairs outside the GEC canteen. It was lunchtime and people were milling around when I started to feel quite strange, confused and unwell. The next thing I knew, *bang, drop*, I collapsed and fell down the stairs.

When I came to, I was vomiting, and three people were

standing over me looking concerned. One of them was my boss, John Heightley, who called an ambulance. When we got to St Cross, the doctors assessed me but didn't know for sure what had happened. There was speculation around whether I'd had a fit or passed out, or possibly just lost my footing. In the end they concluded I was fine and told me if it happened again I should seek emergency help.

And happen again it did. Luckily Pat was there this time, and it was obvious to her, with her medical knowledge, I was having a seizure. We were walking down the road near GEC and I saw a person I thought I recognised coming towards me.

'Where do I know her from?' I said to Pat. The next minute I started to feel that same funny, confused feeling I'd had before, so we sat down on a bench.

Pat was talking to me but I didn't reply. I was completely out of it. She told me afterwards that my head had rolled around to my left and she couldn't see my face. She thought something was off, so she got up and walked around me, examining me, and realised I was having a seizure. She knew she needed to call an ambulance, but she didn't want to leave me. Luckily, there was a phone box across the road with a man standing beside it. Pat shouted out to him, 'Quick – can you phone for an ambulance, please?' The man went into the phone box and then came straight back out and yelled, 'What's the number?'

Pat thought that was weird, since everybody knows the emergency services number.

'999,' she called out.

The man quickly called the ambulance and then crossed the road. 'Is he okay?' he asked. 'I'm a doctor from Italy, and I've just arrived to work at the local hospital.'

What were the odds? It certainly explained why he didn't know the emergency services number. He kindly stayed with Pat until the ambulance arrived. In the meantime, a small crowd had formed, offering their helpful advice as I continued to seize away. 'Stick a spoon in his mouth,' they told Pat and the doctor. Pat's response was, 'You wouldn't want to stick a spoon in someone's mouth when they're having a seizure, mate. That would be a good way to lose a spoon.'

This time the ambulance took me to St Cross again. Ultimately, they diagnosed me with epilepsy, brought on by the operation and the clots on the brain. Apparently, it can take up to eighteen months for somebody who has had a stroke to develop seizures.

Normally with epilepsy, it's flashing lights that trigger it. In my case, for whatever reason, it was when I saw somebody I thought I recognised, and my brain experienced conflict in trying to work out how I knew them. Did I work with them? Was I at school with them? Whatever it was, it was too much for my brain and then, *boof*, it short-circuited.

Pat came with me in the ambulance to St Cross. While I was in casualty and still very groggy, a doctor said, 'Of course, this could well be an extension of the AVM up into his brain. I don't know that they'll be able to do anything for him.' Pat was appalled by this throwaway diagnosis, thinking I might die and she'd not even had the chance to marry the man of her dreams. So she phoned Professor Allison at the Hammersmith and told him what the doctor had said.

He reassured her there was no way the AVM could extend up into the brain. 'I know the scans inside out, upside down, and round and round. He would've seized because of the stroke,' he said.

'Oh, thank God for that,' said Pat.

'I'll sort out a neurologist and I'll give you the name,' said Professor Allison. 'Just get your GP to write a referral.'

When we were at the Hammersmith to see the neurologist and have some scans done, I mentioned I was concerned I might have a seizure on my wedding day because there would be guests I hadn't seen for a number of years, and my brain might have a complete meltdown as I tried to process where they fit into my life. He laughed and said, 'You'll be fine – we'll have you on medication by then and I'm sure you'll be in control.'

The medication did work in time, but initially it made me very tired, and I kept falling asleep, so they adjusted the dosage until it felt right. I wasn't allowed to drive for a couple of years. Pat was always the designated driver, whether we were going to work or out for dinner, and she would say, 'After these two years are up, Jerry, *you* are driving everywhere, and *I'm* going to have a few drinks!'

CHAPTER 15

Wedding Bells and a Brush with Fame

It was the night before the wedding and we'd taken the vicar up on his kind offer to stay at the vicarage. When he asked us what our normal sleeping arrangements were, we told him we slept in the same bed together. 'Okay, then, you can have my bed and I'll sleep in the spare room,' he said.

That night I lay in bed, staring up at the big black crucifix above the headboard, thinking, '*Lord Jesus Christ, forgive me for what we are doing sleeping together in the vicar's bed the night before we get married. Bless me, Father, for I have sinned.*'

The next morning dawned – Saturday, 15 August 1992. My family joined us at the vicar's house to help get things ready for the wedding. Mum even got the ironing board out and ironed the vicar's white liturgical vestments for him. We were anticipating a day full of joy and happiness, and the weather was perfect – even though the weather had been awful the previous day.

I dressed up in a kilt, as did three other Scotsmen who'd also done the graduate training at GEC in Rugby. My kilt was red and green Stewart tartan since my grandmother was a Stewart. We kilt-wearing gentlemen and Steve Rigg, my best man, met at the Dorset Arms, a classic old village pub across the road from the church. We indulged in some fine Scottish whisky before heading across the road to St Swithun's. As we climbed the hill towards the big stone church, the impressive stone clock tower showed it was just after 1:30pm. The guests would soon arrive for the wedding at 2pm.

As the guests poured into the church, they were told to sit wherever they wanted, rather than doing the traditional thing of one side for the bride and one for the groom. We didn't want it to look asymmetrical as Pat had fewer guests on the list than I did after what had happened with her family and her brother. But her cousins and friends from the hospital came.

It was a bit tricky for my best man and photographer, Steve, who had to wait outside the church to take pictures of Pat as she arrived. Once he'd photographed her getting out of the car and entering the vestibule, he had to hightail it down the side of the church to stand beside me near the altar and capture her walking down the aisle towards us with George, who had agreed to give her away in the absence of her own father. Steve was also the keeper of the wedding rings, so his role was quite a large one in the proceedings.

As the strains of Richard Wagner's 'Bridal Chorus' rang out, the guests all craned their necks to get a look at the bride. The massive organ echoed throughout the old church, which had been built in 1789, though there had been a church on the site since the eleventh century. It was such an enormous church that it took quite some time for Pat to make it down the aisle.

She was wearing a beautiful cream wedding dress. Her mother had insisted on cream, not white, which was one thing Pat was fine with since she claimed she looked horrible in white. It was a floor-length dress, fitted and off-the-shoulder, with a detachable train she could remove later. She had a veil over her face and her long hair worn up.

My sister, Sharon, was her bridesmaid, in a peach and cream, off-the-shoulder, knee-length number that Pat had made to save money. Stephen was our page boy, all dressed up in a little suit we'd had tailored for him.

It was an Anglican ceremony, even though I'd been brought up Catholic. I suppose you could say I was lapsed by that stage, as I hadn't been to church for a very long time. And St Swithun's was an inclusive church that welcomed people of any religion.

Pat quickly noticed there were a couple of interlopers in the congregation and whispered to me to have a look up the back of the church. We figured Pat's parents had sent some spies. There were four of them and they hadn't been invited to the wedding, but Pat knew vaguely who they were.

After we had first told Father Richard what had happened, he had gone to see Pat's parents. He knocked on the door and informed them the wedding was definitely going ahead, but there was no expectation they should come under the circumstances. Just in case they had any intention of turning up to the wedding and raising their hand when the priest said, '… if anyone has any objections to this holy matrimony, speak now or forever hold your peace.'

But now that these interlopers were in the church, I was a little paranoid. What if they were here on behalf of Pat's parents and planned to object? Spies at the back of the church – just what you don't need on your wedding day…

Happily, that didn't happen and the wedding ceremony itself went off without a hitch. We signed the paperwork, and Mr and

Mrs Morrissey walked down the aisle together as the crowd cheered and clapped.

East Court Mansion was close to St Swithun's, so it was a quick trip there to meet the rest of our guests who were not at the church but had been invited to the reception. We literally paid just a few pounds per head and not only was it the cheapest wedding reception you could imagine, it was also the best. The only thing that really mattered was that we were together, married and sharing the experience with all the people we loved.

I remember saying to George that night how pleased I was he had given Pat away and that I considered him to be my father. I told him that over the years he'd acted more like my father than my own, and he'd been as committed to me and Sharon as he had to his own son, Paul. We were two kids from a kind of war zone and he'd handled all the baggage that came with that so well. I don't think I'd ever told him how much I appreciated the support he'd been to my mother as well, throughout everything I'd been through, so it felt like on my wedding day, I wanted him to know, without a shadow of a doubt, that he *was* my father.

At the end of the night, my mother and several other willing guests stayed to clean the crockery and the glasses, while Pat and I departed for a night at the White Horse.

The next day, Steve Cook had organised a chauffeur-driven car to take us to the airport and another to pick us up when we arrived in Vienna. He'd booked the best room at Vienna's K+K Palais Hotel for us. It was the honeymoon of a lifetime … so good we repeated it again twenty-five years later and stayed in that same room.

~

When Pat first moved up to Rugby, she was doing the agency work and I was still on a pittance as a graduate trainee so we didn't have a lot of money. We'd saved for a deposit to rent a house and gathered up some hand-me-down furniture from friends and family. Up until that point, I'd been staying with Richard Drabble, but that wasn't really the place for Pat and Stephen, so we'd found our own first place together.

Pat was doing a lot of night shifts and she often bought *Take a Break* to keep herself awake during her breaks, even though I'd tease her about reading trashy magazines. She'd say, 'Well, you try reading a book in the wee small hours of the morning and staying awake!'

One day she said, 'Look, Jerry, they're giving away 250 pounds for real-life stories in *Take a Break*.'

'Wow, 250 pounds?' My brain was starting to whirr … 250 pounds was a lot of money in those days.

'No, Jerry, you can't…' said Pat, reading my mind.

Despite her reservations, when she went off to work that night, I wrote down our story about my surgery and her nursing me back to health, and sent it off to *Take a Break*. A few weeks later we received a phone call – they wanted to feature us in the magazine. They sent a journalist and photographer to our house along with a cheque for 250 pounds.

That was the beginning of our notoriety. A few years later, we got a call from a TV show called *The Big Breakfast*, hosted by Chris Evans, a carrot-topped presenter who was a big deal in the UK at the time. They had obviously been trawling through years' worth of these real-life stories in *Take a Break* and picked up on ours. They paid for us to go to London for the day to pre-record a piece about me being close to death and Pat nursing me back to life. I remember they had us skipping down a cobblestone street, but I don't remember much else about it.

From there, we were invited onto a live chat show called *The Time, The Place* with a presenter called John Stapleton who would roam around the audience and question people. You were led to believe it was a complete coincidence that someone's story fit the theme of the episode. This episode was about being in a relationship that could be considered questionable. With Pat being a nurse and me as her patient, I guess they saw our relationship as one that could be frowned upon. We were placed strategically in the audience and Stapleton just happened to ask us, 'So, what's your story?' We told him briefly and he said, 'Should you have been in a relationship? Is that ethical?'

'Well, it didn't start until he ceased to be a patient and had left the hospital, you know,' said Pat. 'It was all done appropriately.' I'm not sure how impressed she was that my *Take a Break* article had led to this – insinuations being made on national TV about the ethics of us being together.

But I wasn't finished yet. One day, I saw in the local paper they were giving away a free meal on Valentine's Day at the local Italian restaurant and they were calling for romantic stories. So I submitted much the same story I did for *Take a Break* and we won the meal.

Pat was getting calls at the hospital from journalists left, right and centre. The lady on the switchboard told her it was like having a celebrity on staff with having to field all these phone calls from people wanting our story. After that, Pat came after me with a big stick, saying, 'Why have you done this?' She had to ask the switchboard to screen who was calling and, if they were journalists, tell them not to put through any more calls.

~

One good thing that came out of it was meeting Danneka. She was a baby who also had an AVM, and her grandmother had seen our story in *Take a Break*. She recognised me in the street one day, since they also lived in Rugby, and introduced herself. She asked me if I was the guy from *Take a Break* and told me that her granddaughter had the same problem as me.

She explained how worried they were about this little girl. I told her I was happy to have a chat with the family and she gave me her daughter's phone number. That night I phoned her up and Pat and I went around to meet them. The little girl, Danneka, was only about eighteen months old. When we arrived, she was lying on her face in the big bay window and the sun was coming down, so you couldn't see anything. As we sat and talked to her parents, we could hear her waking up and getting a little restless. When her mum went and got her, we saw the AVM. We were shocked. It was huge – much bigger than mine. It was immense.

We asked who they were seeing for treatment and they said a dermatologist. I was sitting there thinking, '*Oh geez, a dermatologist can't help.*' He'd put her on some steroids to try and shrink it, but it was a vascular issue so that wouldn't have worked. I explained to them they really should see a vascular specialist, but it was probably overwhelming for them and they didn't really take it in. We saw them several times after that and kept up to date on the treatment they were getting – there's only so much you can tell people without feeling like you're ramming a point down their throat. I went through, in quite some detail, all the various people I'd seen over the years. But in the end, it was up to them and their doctor, not us, so it was just pure luck what happened next.

It was about a year after we'd met them, and Pat was still doing agency work at St Cross. She was working an early shift on a general surgery ward. When she went for her coffee break, there were some nurses from the children's ward in the lunchroom. Pat heard one of them say, '… and then the blood was just everywhere; it was carnage. This little baby bleeding from her face.' Pat was thinking, 'Surely not – it couldn't be…'

She went past the children's ward after having her coffee, and, sure enough, Danneka's mother, father and grandmother were sitting outside the ward in a terrible state.

Pat raced back to the ward she was on and said to the ward sister, 'Look, I know I've got to get some work done here. But have you heard about the baby?'

'Oh, I've heard about the baby,' she said.

'I know them,' Pat said. 'Perhaps I could be of some assistance because my husband had one of these AVMs and he used to get bleeds just like that.'

The ward sister said she should go, but when Pat got there, it seemed like nobody knew what to do. The consultant paediatrician was in the office with the textbook out; these things were just so rare it wasn't surprising he didn't know what to do.

Pat got a piece of paper and wrote down Brent Tanner's name and number, and Professor Allison's as well. She had their numbers burned into her brain. She told Danneka's parents these two doctors were the people they needed to speak to.

And clearly that's what they did because, years later, Pat did a little Facebook stalking and there she was, Danneka, all grown up with just a little scar on her face. By then the plastic surgeons did laser surgery so it was less invasive and the scar would have faded as she grew up.

It felt good to be able to help someone who was going through the same trauma I'd been through. In fact, the surgeons at the QVH would ask me on occasion to speak to people who came in with an AVM when I was at the hospital for outpatient appointments. I would spend some time with them, counselling them a little about what to expect and helping to allay their fears a little. I liked being able to give back in that way.

CHAPTER 16

Near-Death Encounters of a Different Kind

Over the years following the operation, my body started to reject the pieces of bone that had been inserted into my jaw. Because they were not connected to blood supply, these bits of bone would die; I'd get shards of dead bone coming up from the mandible, and my body would try to push it out through the gum. These horrible little infected lumps would form and then burst, and green pus would shoot out. In the meantime, I'd get high temperatures and feel quite poorly because my body was fighting the infection.

This is why I was pleased I didn't take up the offer from the maxillofacial surgeons to have permanent dental implants to replace all my lower teeth. During the recovery phase after the operation, the surgeons had had a lower set of dentures made to replace all my lower teeth. However, during the fitting process, my gums bled. This was not a major issue, as the life-threatening AVM had been removed. However, my brain was hardwired that every time I tasted blood in my mouth, I thought I would bleed to death. Maybe it had been too early in the recovery process to try dentures, but mentally I couldn't handle the shock that my body would go into and decided that I would just live my life without any bottom teeth.

If I'd had the implants, unless I'd had them removed again, it would have prevented the pieces of dead bone my body was rejecting and wanting to get rid of from being ejected. I also had to be careful because it could even turn into osteomyelitis – a bone infection that could be quite serious.

In time, I had day surgery in London with Colin Hopper, the maxillofacial surgeon. The surgical procedure was called 'debridement', and Colin said, 'It's just like peeling an orange, Jerry. I'll peel the orange, then I'll just take all the dead bone out that I can see. I'll flush it out and then I'll just sew the orange back up.' Maybe these surgeons practise stitching with oranges – who knows?

Otherwise, though, my health was continuing to improve and so was my work situation. By the time I was twenty-seven, I had become one of the youngest project managers at GEC, with most of the other project managers in their forties. It was quite a senior role managing the design, manufacture and construction of a power station, and I got promoted quickly. I liked project management – managing teams and finances – and that combination of money and people, and delivering on the project is what I was good at.

A few years later, I went to work for Rolls-Royce, which is famous for its cars, but it also builds engines for aircraft such as jumbo jets and the large Boeing 777, with fifty-megawatt (MW) twin engines. Rolls-Royce had this novel idea of taking these aircraft engines, sticking them on a base plate, connecting them to a generator and creating a small power station. So I came in as a project manager at the start of this new offshoot Rolls-Royce company, constructing 25–100MW gas-fired power stations producing heat and power to be distributed to the local community. I was also learning more about business development in this role, since I was involved in developing and negotiating on collaboration agreements, and analysing and assessing joint venture and acquisition targets. I also started travelling more – to Japan in particular.

In 1999, I went to work for an American company called PSEG (Public Service Enterprise Group) and I'd commute to London and fly to New York where the company was based. This company was a developer in the energy business. It built new power stations and bought and upgraded old ones, and sold the power on. For example, on and off for eighteen months I did some work in Poland, where we bought old power stations that the Polish government didn't have enough money to invest in. We would go in, do the due diligence, look at all the technical contract conditions, and invest tens of millions of American dollars, upgrading everything. Then we would set up a contract with the government to export the electricity.

I'd always set off the scanning machines in the airport when I travelled – particularly in Turkey, it seemed, since its machines were so dated. I'd take off my belt first and then my shoes. And it would still go off – so I'd point at my face. It was all the spring coils I'd had inserted during the embolisations. After a while, because I was such a frequent traveller, they got to know me and I'd just point to my face and remind them, 'I've got metal bits in here.' Even today, when I get an x-ray, you can actually see the spring coils in my face.

In this role for PSEG, I was dealing with contract conditions at a strategic and commercial development level, making sure that from a business point of view, you could raise the money and get the revenue streams in as well. I was also giving presentations to the board, asking for equity investment, and engaging with international banks to raise debt to fund the construction of these multimillion-dollar power projects. I loved it. It was challenging being responsible for all the technical and commercial aspects of developments, from inception to commercial operation, including alignment of the contractual architecture like shareholder agreements, power purchase agreements, fuel supply, transmission, construction, and operation and maintenance agreements. We had a small but high-performance team working on these complicated deals.

While I was at GEC, I had done an MBA in project management. At Rolls-Royce, I started a law degree part-time to learn more about dealing with contractual terms and conditions. It took me about five years to finish, while I was working and travelling as well, but it certainly helped in my role at PSEG where I was involved with plenty of legal issues.

~

One trip to Turkey for PSEG took place in August 1999. I was in a hotel in Ankara when an earthquake struck in the middle of the night. The epicentre was in Izmir, several hours from Ankara, but it still made our whole hotel shake and the windows rattle. It was a massive disaster, with about 18,000 people killed and 300,000 losing their homes. Total devastation. All telecommunications were down and I couldn't contact Pat, so she was extremely worried about whether I was okay. It was two weeks before we could catch a flight out because all essential services were closed down.

I also flew from Birmingham to Turkey on 11 September 2001. I remember looking at a flight leaving for New York and wishing I was going there instead. We had to change planes in Germany, and that's when I saw the footage of a plane flying into the Twin Towers, but I couldn't grasp what the whole story was – it was all in German. When I got to my hotel in Turkey and called Pat, that's when I found out the full extent of the disaster. She told me about how the Twin Towers had collapsed, killing thousands of people. I told her about seeing the plane at Birmingham Airport and how I wished I'd been flying to New York that day. I couldn't believe what had taken place and was extremely grateful I was in Turkey instead.

~

I have, in fact, been in the proximity of a range of terrorist events and natural disasters, but there's not enough room to go into all of that here. Instead, I will tell you about my time in Italy fraternising with the Mafia. I like to call this phase of my life 'the Italian job'.

I was dealing with renewable energy projects – little baby biomass power stations – in southern Italy over about eighteen months. We'd chop trees down and make wood pellets to fuel the boilers. The Mafia owned all the land, so we had to deal with them indirectly. I said to Pat, 'Look, if I die, it's not suicide, okay? I want the foreign office to investigate my death.' I even went to my managing director, Matthew McGrath, and said, 'Matthew, in Italy, they shoot judges and kill policemen. I think these guys might be in the Mafia.' And he laughed.

'Of course they are,' he said. 'But don't worry about it, Jerry.'

'Why is that?'

'Because you're walking in with like a …' he gestured to his chest with his hands, 'with a big cheque on your chest, right? They just want some of the company's money.'

At that time, the European Union was giving grants to landowners if they got into renewables. You'd get a double reward if you exported renewable electricity, so it was money all around. The Mafia loved this because they owned the land and they were exporting as well.

Down south in the Calabria region, I met this guy, Vincenzo, who was your typical southern Italian – small with jet-black hair. I remember walking down the streets of this little town with him and people scattered. It was like Moses parting the Red Sea. He was my main contact, and he'd take us to the absolute best restaurants in the area. The fish, the wine, the pasta – it was a different world.

He took me to meet one of the big bosses who lived in this baronial castle. I didn't speak much Italian – about forty or fifty words – so I was just chilling, sitting with some of the other guys from my company, having this lovely meal, making pleasantries. The big boss was at the other end of the table with three or four men in suits.

All day we'd been looking at eucalyptus trees on the land because they were ideal for the wood pellets to feed the power station. The next minute, this fly started buzzing around the cupcakes on the table and it was about to land, so I banged the table and made the cupcakes jump. *Boom!* The next thing we knew, the three guys surrounding the boss had each pulled out a gun because they thought they were under threat or being shot at.

After that I thought, '*I've had enough.*' I came back to Pat and said, 'Pat, I can't do this anymore. There must be an easier way to earn a living.' I had an Italian colleague, and I told him the scenario.

'You'll be fine, Jerry,' he said. 'They start off by kneecapping people first.'

~

Yet another life-threatening experience took place in Italy, again thanks to the Mafia. Alberto was our Mafioso Italian rep as he was fluent in English.

He was driving on the highway between our offices in Milan and Rome. It had been raining that day and the road was slippery. The car skidded and Alberto lost control of the car – suddenly we were speeding towards the central reservation. My colleague, Alan Williamson, was in the back seat with me, and this Finnish guy we were doing business with was in the front with Alberto. The Finn was in total panic mode, looking like a meerkat. He thought he was going to go through the windscreen. Everybody dropped into the brace position, except me. I just casually watched the proceedings. Then as the car bounced around and hit the central reservation before rebounding back across into our lane, I calmly removed a pen from my shirt pocket and placed it down at my side.

Afterwards, Alan said to me, 'Why did you do that, with all the madness going on?'

'Alan, the first thing I thought of is: if we have a crash, this pen is going to pierce my chest and go straight through my heart.'

It was one of those moments when time expands and the events of your whole life run through your head – and all the possibilities of the situation too. I just casually picked the pen out of my pocket and put it down. I guess it just shows you the sort of mindset I was in.

I'd already had so many encounters with death that I'd learned to keep cool and think of things logically. When I think back to almost bleeding to death on several occasions and hearing the heart monitor going at 200-odd beats per minute, I actually learned to bring my heart rate down with my own little feedback system. Over the years, I had learned to relax no matter what because I knew the faster my heart was beating, the more blood would pump out.

Every time I have bumped into Alan Williamson over the years, he refers to that story. And in a twist of fate, a few years later, I heard that Alberto did actually die in a car crash.

~

By the early noughties, the American company I worked for, PSEG, was gradually getting smaller and smaller. It was selling power stations and not investing, and then drawing back to the States after selling the assets. I was there right to the very end. And then an opportunity came up to go to Scotland and work on the railways.

The UK railways were in a sorry state in the late nineties. There had been some serious accidents that exposed the stewardship shortcomings of the privatised national railway infrastructure company, Railtrack. Four people were killed and over 70 people injured in a derailment at Hatfield. And in one of the worst rail accidents in British history, thirty-one people were killed and 244 injured when two trains collided due to a signalling error at Ladbroke Grove. Hence, the government began investing money to improve the situation. I equated problems and money with opportunities, so I discussed it with Pat. I'd been in energy since I graduated and the railways seemed like it was the same sort of stuff: safety critical projects in a highly regulated environment, managing teams, plant and machinery, dealing with various forms of contracts, and implementing commercial management strategies.

I applied for a job with Railtrack and was asked to go to London for an interview. When I told the interviewer, also a Scotsman, that I came from Drumchapel, he asked me where I had gone to school. It was a classic test to determine if you were Catholic or Protestant. My heart sank instantly. I thought, '*Oh, here we go. The minute I open my mouth and say, "St Pius Primary and Secondary", the interview will be as good as over.*' What difference does it make what school I attended? What matters is the qualifications I've achieved and my work experience along with my personal skills – that's what should determine my suitability for this job! Turns out I needn't have worried – his son was a ball boy at Celtic Park and he had a season ticket, so, in this case, going to a Catholic school wasn't a problem.

The interview went really well, and I was offered the job, but it was based in Glasgow. When I got back home, I sounded Pat out about whether she'd be interested in moving to Scotland. She hadn't been there before, so I suggested we visit over the next few weekends and have a look around. I would take her to the Drum, show her where I'd grown up and introduce her to the 'culture'.

We drove up and stayed in a little hotel and drove out to Drumchapel. I had a big black Rover 800 series, which was like a drug dealer's car. I took her to Summerhill Road first and then Carolside Drive, and kept the engine running as I pointed out the verandah where I used to hang out as a teenager.

'Switch the engine off, Jerry,' said Pat. 'I want to get out and have a look around.'

'No, we'll just keep the engine running and stay in the car.'

'Why is that?'

'Well, we might need to make a quick getaway because you can't go staring at people up there on the verandahs. They're likely to come down and hit you or throw something at you. This is a war zone, you know. When they see this car and us pointing up at them, they'll think we're undercover police or social security. This is the mindset that you're walking into here, Pat. This isn't a tourist area where you get out and enjoy your surroundings.'

By this point, Pat was starting to take pictures.

'Don't take any pictures,' I said. 'We'll get chibbed!'

Pat looked confused. 'What's that?'

'Stabbed!'

She ignored me, assuming I was making a drama out of nothing, and kept taking pictures of people hanging out on the verandah where I used to live, at number 73 Carolside Drive, so I kept the engine running just in case.

I knew exactly what Glasgow was like, but I wanted Pat to be comfortable with the move. She had come from Canada to East Grinstead – that nice, small English town – and her parents were reasonably well off; she was used to big fancy houses with front and back gardens. Glasgow was something else entirely.

After the 'cultural awareness weekends', Pat said she quite liked Glasgow and didn't mind moving. She liked the fact that if she went into the shops, people spoke to her and held the door open and said 'please' and 'thank you'. We'd have a lot of banter with shop assistants, which she was not used to. In the southeast of England, people are a bit more reserved; you'd be seen as a weirdo if you tried to make conversation with a stranger.

～

We moved to Stewarton in East Ayrshire, about thirty kilometres southwest of Glasgow, in 2003. Stephen had left school and was working in Nottingham by then, so it was just Pat and me. We rented Pheasant Cottage beside the big mansion on Robertland Estate. The eighty-acre estate was owned by Alan Williamson, the guy in the back seat of the car with me on the Italian job. Stewarton was known as 'Bonnet Toun' (town) due to its role in the production of traditional Scottish headwear and ceremonial 'bunnets' for the Scottish regiments stretching back to the 1400s.

We'd sold our house in Rugby, so the plan was to eventually buy a place in Stewarton. This would be the third house we'd purchased together. The house we'd just sold was really quite posh for a boy from the Drum. It was on Elsee Road – one of the most sought-after locations in Rugby – a massive Edwardian house spread over three floors. So we were happy to take our time to find something just as nice in Stewarton.

Pat went looking at houses during the day while I was at work, and she would tell me about them when I got home in the evening. She was very excited about an old manse she'd found, a Victorian villa built for the church in 1874. It sat at the top of a hill so the minister could look down across Stewarton at his flock.

We went to see it together on a Friday afternoon. It was two-storey, with this imposing grand entrance and high ceilings, bay windows, cornices, ceiling roses, and substantial grounds and gardens. As we walked around, we both agreed this was *the* house. In Scotland, they have a sealed bid system for purchasing houses whereby you put your offer in an envelope and the highest bidder is successful.

I said to Pat, 'Look, why don't I say to the owner, "Let's save all the hassle and just give you an offer" and see if he accepts it?'

The owner was there that afternoon, and he accepted our offer on the spot. He liked the fact that we had the money ready to go, and there would be less paperwork involved. Then he offered us a glass of champagne to celebrate, and another, and then some wine. We got so drunk that night, we ended up staying over. The next morning, we got up and thought, '*WTF?*' We'd just bought a house, and we didn't even know the people, yet we'd ended up staying for the night!

The deal went through and we moved in a few weeks later. One day, while we were still unpacking, there was a knock at the door. Pat answered, since I was at work, and found two serious-looking detectives on the doorstep. It seemed they were looking for the previous owners. Pat told them we'd just moved in. It would've been obvious she was telling the truth since she had an English accent and you could see all our boxes piled up in the background. They asked her if she knew where the owners had gone, and she told them they'd immigrated to Spain. They'd packed up their van, taken the two kids and the dog, and left behind their cats, which we'd inherited: Fluffkin and Munchkin.

The detectives didn't tell us why they wanted to speak to the previous owners but we assumed it must have been something serious and maybe that's why he'd done a deal with us so quickly, because he wanted the cash without any technicalities or contracts slowing down the process. Pat gave the detectives their solicitor's contact details, which was all we had to offer. And that's how we became the new owners of the beautiful Ardgowan House.

~

In another twist of fate, while I was working for Railtrack (which then became Network Rail a few months after I started), there was another terrorist event I came close to being involved in.

Following a reorganisation, I was asked to work at King's Cross Station in London, looking after all the big signalling projects that covered London South East. I would fly from Glasgow on a Monday morning and back home on a Friday evening.

On 7 July 2005, as I sat in the office at King's Cross, a bomb exploded in the London Underground beneath me. We were evacuated immediately as thousands of people poured onto the streets of London. There was a constant wail of sirens from police cars, ambulances and fire engines as I walked, in shock, along Euston Road, thinking I would go back to my hotel, the Euston Plaza (now the Hilton Hotel), near Tavistock Square. I stood at the traffic lights on Euston Road, trying to decide whether to turn left into the hotel or right into another Network Rail office and work there for the day. Finally, I decided to turn right and go into the other office … and thank God I did, because just a few minutes later another bomb exploded in a double-decker bus right outside the hotel.

Those London bombings, also referred to as 7/7, were a series of four suicide attacks carried out by Islamic terrorists targeting commuters during the morning rush hour. Fifty-six people died with almost 800 injured. I wandered the streets of London for a few hours and went back to the hotel, but the street was closed off. All my belongings were there, and I had nowhere else to stay since London was in lockdown. No public transport, no communications. I couldn't just go back to my house in Scotland.

As I stood on the street wondering how I could get inside the hotel, I caught the eye of the hotel doorman from behind the police cordon. I had been staying at the hotel Monday to Friday every week for a year by then, and I knew all the staff, as well as their wives' and kids' names, so I had a good relationship with all of them, particularly the doorman. He called me over and took me to the back of the hotel. He let me in through the back entrance and I went up two flights of stairs to my room, where I packed up my suitcase with all of my clothes.

The hotel was being used as a triage station for the injured. Doctors from the British Medical Association, which was situated right across the road, were helping to treat casualties. The day was getting more and more unbelievable. It was like being on the set of a disaster movie, only it was all too real.

The hotel staff made some phone calls on my behalf and managed to find a room at another hotel five kilometres away. Since there was no public transport, I walked the whole way, trying to get my head around what had happened that day. Later, as I lay in my hotel bed, I thought to myself, *'You just never know what is going to happen on any given day.'* Had I decided to turn left at the traffic lights rather than right that day, I could have walked straight into that double-decker bus exploding.

As the saying goes, 'Tomorrow is promised to no one.' It was yet another reminder for me to make the most of every moment.

CHAPTER 17

The Irish Connection

Early one Sunday morning at our house in Stewarton, when I was still half-asleep, I heard Pat saying, 'Oh nooooo, oh nooooo…' I was immediately concerned and sat bolt upright.

'What is it?' I said. 'What's going on?'

She was reading something from her phone and she kept saying it over and over, 'Oh nooooo, oh nooooo' and then 'Jesus Christ!'

'For God's sake, Pat, tell me what's going on!' I was starting to think someone was dead. A family member must have died overnight. Who could it be? Had anyone been ill recently? Or was it a sudden death?

'I just don't believe this!' said Pat. I was fully awake by now and starting to get frustrated. 'What the fuck is going on, Pat? Tell me!'

'Ummm…' she said. 'I've got a Facebook message from a woman who thinks she's related to you! She thinks she's your half-sister.' She passed the phone to me and I read the message:

> **11 Dec 2016 at 9:27**
>
> Hello Pat, sorry to message you out of the blue but I'm trying to trace some family and think I may be your husband's half-sister. Was wondering if you think it would be ok to contact him? I am looking for a Jeremiah Christopher Paul Morrissey, age 52. I totally understand if you do not reply or think it best not to contact. Many thanks and kind regards, Geraldine

I looked at Pat, completely puzzled by this. What half-sister? What was this woman going on about?

Pat explained she'd got the message the day before, but hadn't opened it. We had a friend named Geraldine with a very similar surname to this woman, so she assumed our friend had been hacked. But since she'd woken before me that morning, she'd picked up her phone and decided to have a proper look at it.

I wondered if it was some sort of scam too, but what benefit would anyone gain from claiming to be related to me? My head was spinning, and I didn't know what to think. It was all a bit too much early on a Sunday morning.

'Look, well ... I don't know. I guess we'll get back to her ... but right now, I just need some time to think about it. Let's get some breakfast and work out what to do next.'

I wanted to contact my sister, Sharon, to share what Geraldine had said and discuss the next steps. I was thinking, '*If it is true, then where's it going to lead?*' For forty-odd years, I'd always just thought of Sharon and Paul as my siblings. I was trying to fast-forward my thought process: Could this be a good thing – a happy thing? Or would it just open up a can of worms?

Over a traditional Scottish fry-up of square sausages, fried eggs, Ayrshire bacon, tattie scones, haggis and Stornoway black pudding, I said to Pat, 'First we need to verify things. How about you respond to her message and ask her some questions to see what she knows about Big Jerry?'

Pat agreed, so we made a list of a few basic questions like middle names, dates, the name of Big Jerry's brother, things like that, and sent off the list that afternoon.

Geraldine responded overnight and we read her answers over coffee in the morning. They rang quite true: the timing was right,

178

as were the names we asked her for … it all checked out. I suggested we should speak on the phone the following weekend. On the Sunday evening, I gave her a call. We ended up chatting on the phone for two or three hours, then did it again the following week.

Turns out Big Jerry *did* have another family in Dublin. There were four kids – my half-siblings. Caroline was the oldest. She was in her forties, so she must have been born just after he left us. That would have been the reason he'd done a runner and never come back – he was busy starting this other family in Dublin. Geraldine was the second child, and there were two younger ones, another girl and a boy.

What I really wanted to know straight up was what kind of dad he had been, but I had to be sensitive as we were just getting to know each other. I was quite polite to start, then found myself broaching it by saying, 'He wasn't a good husband or father to us. Hopefully, he was better when he moved from Glasgow to Dublin…?'

'Well, no, he wasn't,' she said, quite matter-of-factly. And that's when it all came out that Geraldine's mother was just as bad as him. There had been no protection from his violent ways at all. It sounded even worse than what we'd had to deal with. At least we'd had Mum looking out for us.

Big Jerry used the divide-and-conquer technique with the four kids as well, and, consequently, they were not close as adults. The third child had fled to Australia, having left home as soon as she could, while the youngest child, a boy, remained close to his parents.

Caroline and her husband came to visit us in Stewarton one weekend. They stayed in a local hotel and brought four of their five kids with them. She had a heart of gold and was so pleased to meet Pat and me. She told us she still struggled mentally from the trauma of her childhood.

When I first spoke to Geraldine, I asked her how she had found out about us. She told us that Big Jerry had been in a nursing home following a couple of strokes. Knowing that his days were probably numbered, Geraldine had asked him outright: 'There's always been a rumour in the family that you've got another family in Glasgow. Is there any truth to it?'

She told us there had been a picture of me and Sharon on the mantlepiece at our grandparents' place, but it was never really discussed. Geraldine also told me that every time her parents had an argument, her mother would shout at Big Jerry: 'Why don't you just fuck off back to your family in Glasgow then...' That's how they knew without really *knowing* for sure.

Big Jerry had confirmed that it was true and Geraldine went on to ask him some questions and take down some notes. *Who did you marry?* Margaret Rose (my mum's name). *What were the kids' names?* Jeremiah and Sharon. *What years were they born?* And so on...

From there, Geraldine did a bit of investigating online, looking for the Morrisseys in Glasgow, Scotland who were the right ages. That's how she found me – and on Facebook she saw that Pat was my wife. She'd decided to contact Pat first ... in case I was like him.

Over forty years later, we had actually found out what had become of Big Jerry. Since he left us, there had been no contact whatsoever, which was just fine with me. Meeting his other children made me think of the ripple effect through the generations and the detrimental impact that just one man can have. I escaped inheriting the same traits as him – or suffering mentally as Caroline had. Some of my half-siblings' kids will probably escape it and have good lives and some of them probably won't. Sometimes people choose to be completely different to the generation before them, and others are just consumed by it and can't escape. They become a victim of it because they can't get the effects of it out of their head.

It's difficult to pass judgement on anyone else in a situation like that because you're not in their head space, but sometimes you've got to ask yourself: Do you want to be the victor or the victim? You need to decide which direction to take and help yourself or get help from others, because you know you're looking at a downward spiral otherwise. If you've got some sort of medical condition where you're not in full possession of your faculties, that's one thing. But if you know you're doing bad things and you do them deliberately anyway, that's monstrous. That was Big Jerry.

After Caroline had visited us in Stewarton, Pat and I went to Dublin to meet Geraldine and her family. Big Jerry died soon after telling Geraldine about us, and I went to see his grave while we were there. He was buried with his parents, my grandparents, up on this little hill, looking down over Dublin. With the sun coming up, I thought it was a nice resting place for someone who had caused so much grief to so many people. Did someone who was just bad through and through deserve to be buried in such a pretty, peaceful place? At least he was underground and couldn't do any more harm to anyone ever again.

CHAPTER 18

It's Now or Never

We had been trying to have a baby for years. Pat first became pregnant not long after we were married and we were so excited. But within a few weeks, she was experiencing some spotting, so we booked her in for an early scan. As she was lying on the table, Pat noticed the look on the sonographer's face and knew immediately something was wrong. The sonographer disappeared to fetch the doctor, who came in and said, 'I'm sorry, it's not good news. There's nothing there. You must have miscarried when you had the spotting.' It was a bit of a shock for us both ... and it was just the beginning.

After that first miscarriage, Pat visited our GP. He told her that he would not refer her to a gynaecologist until she had three miscarriages. He sat there at his big leather-topped desk, swivelling in his fancy leather chair, and made light of the situation. He said there might have been an issue with the foetus and that's why she miscarried. Pat was beside herself thinking she had some sort of deformed monster growing inside her; she was distraught and in tears. When Pat told me about it, I thought, 'W*hat a pompous, self-entitled, self-absorbed asshole – what a cheek calling yourself a doctor.*' Pat miscarried again and again, and was finally referred for infertility treatment after the third miscarriage.

The hospital gynaecologist said Pat had been left so long

without treatment (three years) that it was a race against time, as with each passing year she was getting older and fertility starts to decline with age. With a sense of urgency, she started to have all sorts of investigations: bloods, scans, tubal patency to test the fallopian tubes, and so on.

The first approach was IUI (intrauterine insemination), which involved Pat taking a drug called Clomid to increase egg production. It caused some horrendous side effects, including anxiety and panic attacks. The result? No pregnancy. The next level up was IVF (in vitro fertilisation), which involves an egg combined with sperm in vitro – a Latin term meaning 'in glass'.

When she was waiting to have the first round of IVF, she came into the bedroom one morning doubled over in pain. She disappeared into the toilet and when she eventually emerged, she looked distraught. 'There's a baby in the toilet, Jerry,' she said, hysterically. 'I think it's a baby in the toilet!'

When I went to have a look, I could see the outline of what looked like a small foetus in a baggy sack, so we scooped it out and gently put it in a plastic box to take to the pathology lab to have tested, but the results were inconclusive. They weren't really sure what it was – it might have been a baby or it might not. It was a horrific experience all round, though, especially for Pat.

She was injecting herself with medications and hormones for the IVF treatment, which meant she had a lot more hormones pumping through her body, leaving her bloated, irritable and extremely emotional. It was a living nightmare for Pat, but we continued. Twelve eggs were collected, eight good viable ones, but no fertilisation took place. We were shattered. We had also used up all our savings and had to take out a bank loan to further fund the treatment.

Cranking it up to the next level, we tried ICSI (intracytoplasmic sperm injection), which involved injecting my sperm into Pat's eggs in the laboratory. Of six eggs, three were viable and yet there was zero implantation. The physical and emotional pain that Pat experienced, and the knock-on effect for me as well, in losing children we already loved and never got to meet, was unbearable. I had already given our children names like Rebecca and Rachel. I had their lives already mapped out.

After that we decided to call it a day. It was too much, over and over – the disappointment, the stress on Pat's body. At one point, I didn't think we would ever get over the trauma, and I admit it took years for us to recover.

A few months after we first moved to Scotland, Pat found out she was pregnant. Out of the blue. No IVF treatment, it just happened naturally. Would this be the pregnancy that would go to full term? One Saturday morning, Pat woke up in intractable pain. We quickly jumped in the car and drove to an emergency obstetrics clinic where we were kept waiting. I watched as the colour slowly drained from her face. The fact that she was bleeding internally was only picked up when the medical staff scanned her, at which point they were extremely apologetic. It was an ectopic pregnancy and Pat's life was in danger. She needed emergency surgery.

As they wheeled her into the operating theatre, she said, 'Jerry, I think you better contact my mother.' We hadn't spoken to Rosemary since the day she threw us out of her house before the wedding more than ten years earlier. I called and told her that Pat had had an ectopic pregnancy and time was of the essence as she had internal bleeding. In fairness to Rosemary, she realised the magnitude of the situation and was polite and concerned.

She followed up the phone call by sending flowers to Pat in the hospital, which was a nice touch appreciated by us both.

I couldn't believe what was happening to Pat. The thought of losing her in an attempt to have a child was not worth it in my mind. That was a price I couldn't afford to pay. After Pat went into the operating theatre, I wasn't too sure what to do with myself. My head was bursting at the thought of losing her and possibly never seeing her again. I walked back to our car in the hospital car park and sat there alone, overcome with immense sadness. I was absolutely gutted. I felt as if someone had come along and ripped my heart straight out of my body while I was still alive. It was a horrible feeling. Tears slowly rolled down my face. There was no one around, no one saw me, and I made no noise – no wailing, no whimpering, nothing. Just tears rolling steadily down my face.

As a child, I had learned to cry silently under my bedcovers as Big Jerry dished out beatings to my mum. I couldn't risk him hearing. I guess it was my self-protection mechanism, shielding me from hurt and pain. I have always just noted my emotions and then neatly stored and locked them away in a box in my mind. But when the pain becomes so unbearable, as it did on that day, the emotions need to come out. I just sat there in the car with tears flowing down my face in absolute silence.

Thank God Pat survived the operation, and after a blood transfusion and a few days in hospital, she returned home. She recovered well and, after a few months, was back to normal health … at least for the moment.

~

As a fitness challenge, in 2007, we were preparing to do a six-day walk called the West Highland Way, which is 155 kilometres from Milngavie to Fort William, so we'd been covering a lot of miles to get fit. We thought it was just tiredness from all the walking, but Pat would trip over and fall randomly. She also had a problem with her eyes and bad headaches, as well as other little symptoms that didn't quite add up.

When we still lived in Rugby, Pat had noticed a strange numbness creeping up from her hands to her armpits and from her feet up to her chest. She went to the GP, and he told her it was probably post-viral symptoms and to come back in a couple of weeks if it was no better. It did improve, but she still had terrible pins and needles in her hands, so it was back to the GP again.

This time he referred her to a neurologist, who told her it sounded like multiple sclerosis (MS). 'But,' he said, 'you're too old at thirty-four to be presenting with MS.' Pat thought, *'Oh well, that's good then!'* and put it to the back of her mind. He sent her off for some nerve tests, but the results came back normal. We were planning to move to Scotland around then, and, since she seemed to be doing okay, she didn't bother following up on it further.

In fact, Pat had been fourteen or fifteen when she first started noticing numbness and tingling. She would notice the tip of her nose being numb and feel like she'd had an injection from the dentist. Also around that time, she recalls being on an adventure weekend where there was a climbing wall and she didn't seem to be able to rely on her left leg to support her weight, which made her stumble. It just seemed unusual to her at the time, with all the other kids climbing like monkeys.

When she finally *was* diagnosed with MS in Scotland in 2007, after the creeping numbness presented itself again, it was by her

GP. He told her he'd seen many people with the disorder and sent her off to a neurologist for an MRI scan. The neurologist showed us the scan and told us it was bad news, as he pointed to the small white spots on the brain and spinal cord that looked like little stars in the black sky. He explained that was where the sheath that covers the nerve was exposed.

Although it certainly was bad news, in some ways, the diagnosis was a relief because we were starting to think it was a brain tumour or something just as sinister causing these idiosyncrasies. We figured at least MS would give us some time, whereas if it was a brain tumour, she might not have long at all. After the diagnosis, Pat's physical condition slowly deteriorated. She had a relapse, more falls and then developed foot drop, which makes lifting the front part of the foot difficult, after walking for only about 100 metres. That's when she started to use a walking stick to get about.

The MS physiotherapist gave her a FES (functional electrical stimulation) machine with electrodes that attached to her leg. The machine used electrical impulses to stimulate the muscles and cause them to contract. It significantly improved her ability to carry out functional activities such as walking. She developed a mindset based on what she had experienced with me when I had to learn to function all over again after my operation. She would say to me, 'How can I expect you to feel sympathy for me if I am not prepared to put in the hard work that you did after your strokes?'

We bought a treadmill so she could practise walking; having the support and stability of the treadmill guide rails gave her the confidence to walk. It also had a safety key that could be pulled to automatically switch off in case of an emergency. The safety key clipped onto Pat's clothes so the machine would stop if she fell. We also hired a personal trainer who came to our house to do one-on-one sessions focused on Pilates, mobility and strength exercises. After many months of focusing on what she could do, and building her strength and mobility, Pat was no longer falling over. I remember the day we walked in to see the physiotherapist, handed back the FES machine, and Pat said, 'Thanks, but I don't need this anymore.' The physiotherapist was shocked that someone with MS had improved so much they didn't need it. It was a great day.

~

Many years later, when we visited a new MS clinic in Australia, the doctor told Pat she'd been skimming through her past medical history and could see that she'd had quite a number of miscarriages and infertility problems. Pat confirmed this was true, and the doctor went on to explain that, just recently, they'd discovered some people with MS carry an antibody that prevents them from carrying to term. Pat told me she felt so much better after hearing that because there had always been a voice in the back of her head saying, 'If only I'd continued with the IVF, if only I'd continued...' And now she knew it would have been a waste of time. Those eggs just didn't want to be fertilised.

Pat's mother had also had a long period of infertility, which was another thing Pat always used to tell the doctors. It had been nine years between her and her brother. In fact, her parents had looked into adoption. Now, with hindsight, Pat suspects her mother had MS too, since she would fall over all the time. She also had restless foot syndrome and couldn't keep her feet still, plus she was a big list maker, which is a good cover for forgetfulness – another MS symptom.

Pat's only experience with MS otherwise was caring for people as a nurse. There was a guy at the QVH who had been there for two whole years, and he had five pressure sores you could fit a fist in. He wasn't able to walk, and he was emaciated as it was impossible for him to maintain sufficient nutrition. He was 'topped up' with a naso-gastric feed like I'd had post-operation. Pat said if that was going to happen to her, ending up in a wheelchair unable to care for herself, she didn't want to live at that point. She was thinking of how she would take her own life. Would she take an overdose? She didn't want to ask me to assist in her suicide. How long would it be before she was bed bound? She had so many questions. I understood where Pat was coming from and I knew I would feel the same. But I'm happy to say most people wouldn't even pick that she has MS today. She manages it well and is at the gym every day, doing yoga and all the things she possibly can to take care of herself.

But those discussions did create a line of thought in my mind. As far as I was concerned, it was time to travel and see the world, to live for the moment, since who knew how much longer we would have our health and strength and the ability to move around freely.

When I was working at GEC, an older guy there, Noel Thompson, who was close to retirement, had lost his wife. He told me both he and his wife had been working since the age of fourteen. They'd been together since that age too. They were planning to spend some time travelling when they retired. But then, just in his last few months at GEC, Noel's wife had a massive heart attack.

One day I was walking down the street with him at lunchtime and I said, 'Noel, I don't know how you're coping with this, to be honest. Ever since you've been kids, you've been working, and just when you were looking forward to retiring and travelling the world, this happens.'

Well,' Noel said, 'I just try to remember all the good times we had. That's what gets me through.'

People in his generation left school and went straight to work. They didn't go to university unless their family had money. I thought, '*Christ, both of them have been working hard all their lives; they've finally got the end-lap in sight to spend some quality years together, and then it's just gone.*'

The lesson I took from that is, it's fine to have plans for the future but don't neglect the present. It was a reminder for me not to live in the future or the past. There's always that balance of living in the present but planning for the future, of course. But they're not mutually exclusive. The trick is not to neglect living in the present.

What with Noel's experience, all of my own near-death encounters and now Pat's diagnosis, it was time to make some plans for us. '*Don't wait until you're too old to do what you want,*' I told myself.

CHAPTER 19

Life Down Under

In 2012, I spent three months in Perth, Australia, on a work assignment. When I came back to Scotland I said to Pat, 'Australia is such a beautiful place – the climate, the quality of life, even the wide roads. I'd really like to go back one day and see more of it.' For the time being, I put it on the back burner. But in 2015, Pat and I took a three-week holiday to Australia. We visited Melbourne, Sydney, Brisbane and the Whitsundays, where we stayed on an island so tiny we were the only guests there. When we got back to the UK, for the next six months Pat seemed quite depressed being back in the cold climate of Scotland; she'd loved Australia so much.

One evening, we were sitting in a pub in Stewarton, sketching out our plans for our future life together. 'Unfortunately,' I said to Pat, 'we're too old to get accepted in Australia for permanent residency. How about we take a year out and travel around Australia instead?' That's when we started planning our 'gap year' – just like teenagers do between school and university. It would be our middle-age gap year.

I was finishing up a contract in Northern Scotland where I was working on an assignment on the decommissioning of nuclear waste – some of the most radioactive materials on the planet, so really quite dangerous. I'd spent decades working in challenging roles, managing the delivery of major projects in safety critical environments. And since I was working away from home and only got back to see Pat every other weekend, I'd made the most of my time away from home by doing a distance-learning part-time Master of Laws (LLM) in construction law and arbitration – my fourth degree, for which I was most happy to receive a distinction. It was definitely time to take a break and follow up on that impulse to make the most of our time while we were still physically capable.

And so, at the end of January 2018, Pat and I flew into Melbourne and hired a campervan with a toilet/shower like a vertical Formica coffin. Throughout our entire married life, we had not spent a single night in any sort of campervan. I watched YouTube videos about how to connect fresh water and wastewater pipes, and connect the electrics, among other things. Plus it was a steep learning curve getting to grips with driving the van. Luckily for us, in both Australia and the UK you drive on the left-hand side of the road so at least that was one less thing to worry about.

For the whole year we had one holdall-type bag and one rucksack each. In fact, we only travelled with what I could physically carry because I carried Pat's bags too. At the end of the year, I said to Pat, 'We've survived a whole year with only the stuff that I could carry on my back. It just shows you don't need lots of material items to live.' Later, when we went back to our house in Scotland, I said, 'Do we really need all these ornaments? What function or added value are they giving us in life? Do we need them?' And that was well before that documentary on Netflix started a whole movement towards minimalism.

Over the next twelve months, we covered tens of thousands of kilometres around the coast and through the centre of Australia in this campervan, as well as staying in tents, motels, hotels and Airbnbs.

Each day of every week of every month of the entire year, we did something different. We tried to do things outside our comfort zone. We swam naked in a river in the Snowy Mountains; rode on the back of a Harley-Davidson for nine hours around the Mornington Peninsula; and stood on dinosaur footprints over 120 million years old outside Broome. Only Pat was brave enough to jump out of a plane in Byron Bay and thank God her parachute opened; my thinking was, 'Who in their right mind would throw themselves out of a perfectly functional aircraft?' We got up close and personal with crocodiles; visited Albany and the place where the ANZAC fleet left Australia in 1914 to fight in Gallipoli; swam in the hot springs at Mataranka; watched as wild horses emerged from the early morning mist on the banks of the Yellow Water in Kakadu; crossed the Nullarbor Plain ... the list goes on.

One of my favourite memories is the pure wonder of looking up to the southern sky night after night in the outback and seeing the Milky Way with stars twinkling like diamonds against black velvet.

Another highlight was visiting Cape York, the most northern point in Australia. It's a very beautiful place up there in North Queensland where the Great Barrier Reef meets the Daintree Rainforest. However, it was a difficult day for Pat, who struggled with the humidity and the last kilometre, which involved scrambling over rocks. The sweat was dripping off us by the time we got there. At one point I thought I was going to have to carry Pat ... but we got there in the end and took a little picture of ourselves to commemorate it – one of the 49,808 pictures we took that year.

The whole year was superb, well worth the sacrifice of saving lots of money and taking a year out from your career. When we took a trip on The Ghan – the train that runs between Adelaide and Darwin, right through the heart of Australia – there were some elderly people with walking frames. Fair play to them for getting out there. But when we stopped in Coober Pedy, there was an old underground Serbian church and they couldn't get the walking frames down there, so they had to miss out. I said to Pat, 'I'm so pleased we're doing this now when both of us are still physically capable.'

On our first night on The Ghan, we got to know the fifteen or so other travellers in our carriage rather well, and spent the next three nights dancing and singing. When the staff went to bed, we had an open bar until the wee small hours, drinking vast amounts of champagne. In fact, we drank so much champagne, we consumed the entire stock. When the train stopped at Alice Springs, more champagne had to be brought on board.

Even on the quiet days we'd visit museums and art galleries, and cover kilometres walking up and down the floors in those places. Being reasonably fit to make the most of our time that year was necessary. And you just don't know what tomorrow will bring regarding your mobility or your health, so I'm so glad we did it when we did.

~

Early on in our travels, I looked on LinkedIn because I knew some former colleagues were living and working in Australia, and I thought it might be nice to catch up. Richard and Hugh had been my project managers at Network Rail in Scotland and they were working together in Sydney.

I called them and told them we were travelling around Australia and said it'd be great to catch up, so when we were in Sydney we organised to meet them for a bite to eat. It had been fifteen or twenty years since we'd worked together, so it was great to catch up with them and hear about what they were up to these days. They'd both had senior positions in a big construction company, but a few years ago they'd left and set up their own infrastructure consultancy company. Before we left, they asked me if I'd ever thought of working in Sydney. 'I'd love to,' I said, laughing. 'But I really think I'm far too old for them to let me!'

'Actually, that's not the case,' said Hugh. 'If we sponsored you, we could get you a visa for four years. Doesn't matter what age you are. And with a four-year visa you can apply for permanent residency after three years.'

Wow, so it was possible after all. Pat and I were elated to hear this, but we still had a round trip of Australia to complete, so we told the fellows we'd check in with them later in the year when we'd finished our trip.

When we returned at the start of 2019, I said, 'Now, are you guys serious? Because when we go back to Scotland we're going to pack up our belongings, wait for our visa and then we're coming back.'

'We're absolutely serious, Jerry,' said Richard. 'We'll pay for the visa.'

A few weeks later, we flew back to Scotland to pack up and wait for the visa to land. We spent the time getting the house ready to rent out, painting it throughout and meeting all the legal obligations as landlords, like getting the fire alarms linked to the electrical supply.

By May we were back in Sydney, four-year visa in hand, ready to start a whole new phase of life Down Under.

~

For three years, I worked in Sydney as a project director for Hugh and Richard's infrastructure company, working on complex projects and major business change initiatives. After those three years, I could apply for permanent residency.

During this time in Sydney, I had a few health scares. I had been on epilepsy medication for thirty years since the stroke. However, perhaps because of the cumulative impact of taking this medication, it started to have an impact on my blood chemistry. My poor liver had been working so hard to detox all the medications over decades that my body was struggling. I found a neurologist and, over a period of seven months, in a safe and controlled manner, I decreased my medication week by week, aiming to come off it completely.

At the end of the seven months, I had an electroencephalogram (EEG) after my brain had been deliberately stressed. To achieve that end, I was sleep deprived all night. Now, let me tell you, sleep deprivation is a form of torture. Rather than just sit there all night staring into space, I arranged thirty-minute back-to-back Facebook Messenger calls with family and friends from the Northern Hemisphere throughout the night. They were about ten hours behind Sydney time and it was their late afternoon. In the morning, I successfully passed the neurologist's stress tests. For the first time in thirty years, I was epilepsy free and no longer on any sort of medication.

Another unplanned medical drama unfolded in Sydney when I

noticed two small lumps on my chest. I went to the GP, and he sent me for a chest x-ray. I couldn't believe it when I saw the x-ray. You could see the six wires that had been holding my chest together since the heart-lung bypass; two of them had unravelled and were protruding out of my chest. I was referred to a cardiothoracic surgeon who I saw on a Tuesday morning, and by the Friday morning I was under the knife being operated on. The surgeon tried to remove the two wires, but they wouldn't come out and he ended up trimming them back to the bone so that they would not pierce my chest. He also revised my chest scar because, over the years, the skin was becoming very thin. To do this, the surgeon had to remove about an inch of skin all the way down my chest. After the operation, every time I took a breath, I thought my chest was going to burst open, it was so tight. It took a few months for the skin to stretch and become more elastic, and it was several more months before I could get to the gym and do a bench press.

In between these dramas, we had to navigate a few medical problems that Pat had developed, including having her gall bladder removed and a hip replacement.

We thought that because of our age and Pat's MS, we probably wouldn't get permanent residency, but we applied anyway. Pat's neurologist wrote a letter saying she was stable, because the Australian government wanted to know if we were going to end up costing them. Fair enough, really. The neurologist said you really couldn't predict how Pat's situation would change over time – no one could know, and the past isn't necessarily a good indicator of the future.

I also applied for a global talent visa, usually only open to the likes of sportspeople and musicians. They had just opened a category up for infrastructure people, so I had to get letters of endorsement saying I had a special talent (I'm still trying to work out what that is). In the end, though, this was how we were accepted into Australia as permanent residents. It gave me a great opportunity to walk around the house and say to Pat, 'Look at me – I'm a global talent!'

I had enjoyed working in Sydney with Richard and Hugh. But when the opportunity came up to work on the Melbourne Airport rail link, I jumped at it, as Pat and I had been keen on Melbourne right from the start.

~

Before we moved to Melbourne, we spent six weeks in the UK and Ireland. I hadn't seen my family in nearly four years because of COVID lockdowns and no international travel, and my parents weren't getting any younger, so I was keen to get back and see them.

It was traumatic, though. Mum had developed dementia and didn't recognise me. I had exchanged a number of Facebook messages with her in the months leading up to us going back to the UK. Some of the messages were odd, quite bizarre even – sort of mixed up. For example, one message said, 'I've found my long-lost son.' I ignored it because I thought I would see her shortly anyway, so I didn't read too much into it.

I didn't understand why she was behaving so oddly when we first arrived, and I remember thinking, '*WTF is going on here?*' When I spoke to George and Sharon about it, they said she'd deteriorated rapidly over the last few months. I showed her a picture of us from years gone by and asked her who the people in it were. She recognised herself and when I asked her who she was with, she replied, 'That's my baby boy.' That baby boy was sitting right in front of her and she didn't recognise me now; it was devastating. After everything we'd been through together, the connection between my mum and I had always been one of pure, unconditional love, and it still was, but it broke my heart to see her like this.

During our life, we change schools, jobs, careers and houses, and we can even change our partners, but we can never change our mother. There can be only one woman who carries you in her womb for nine months, cares for you during those early years, and, in my case, puts herself in harm's way to protect you physically and mentally during some very dark days. That woman is your mother.

As we boarded the plane back to Australia, I thought it was unlikely I would see her alive again. The thought was unbearably painful. I felt an emptiness inside of me because I was leaving a part of me behind in the UK. I was leaving behind part of my heart with my mother.

~

The other part of my heart, of course, belongs with Pat, and here we were about to enter another new phase of life in Melbourne, Victoria.

Over the years, Pat and I have often been asked how we manage to have such a successful marriage – what's the secret? Over the last thirty years that we have been together, we have seen so many couples get married, divorced, married again and some divorced a second time. We have also known couples who have been together for over thirty years but you can see they don't really love each other. They're together out of habit or they're waiting for the kids to leave home. Perhaps they're frightened to be on their own or unsure if they will find love again in their lives. Each to their own and no path is the right one. I think it's important to at least be true to yourself, though. You can't kid yourself. You are the one who lays your head on the pillow each night and you need to live with yourself – despite what you tell others. You know your own truth.

The truth for Pat and me is that we give our love unconditionally to each other; we don't hold back and we don't make other things a dependency or a precondition of our love. We give it freely and openly. We may feel a little exposed at times (particularly in the early days of the relationship) but this approach has been reciprocated tenfold – it eventually leads to a relationship that is built on trust. We humans are not mind readers. We need to communicate and discuss (in a sensitive way) how we feel about something, and what makes us happy and what makes us sad, and work through any difficulties.

Pat and I love doing the most ordinary activities together that we consider extraordinary – simply because we can *do* them, so we enjoy it while we can because we know nothing lasts forever. Things that involve our most basic human senses: feeling the sun on your skin, being able to move your body in the way it is designed to move, walking and running, and having freedom from pain. Pain, physical or mental, can suck the energy and life right out of you – I am constantly grateful to be free of pain in this stage of my life, allowing me to enjoy the most basic of human activities.

Sometimes it's as simple as prioritising hugs and cuddles – never underestimate the power of physical contact. Sometimes we don't know what to say, and sometimes no words are necessary. Words can be poorly expressed or inadvertently taken out of context. But you can always have a cuddle. There is no misunderstanding with a cuddle. The intention is always genuine.

This journey has taught me that to truly live my best life, I need to accept and love myself unconditionally. It was a revelation that took some time, but it opened the doors to a world of shared experiences with Pat. I've discovered hidden passions – I've loved learning yoga – and I surround myself with positive people – humans with a kind heart and a good soul – who help me become the best version of myself and who share my values of honesty, integrity, loyalty, authenticity and humour.

I think because both Pat and I have had such issues with our health, we appreciate the small things. Health is wealth, as they say. Our physical and mental wellbeing is far more important than wealth in the realm of life satisfaction. Money is great, and I appreciate the fact that I have been able to make a good living through the work I do, but good health is essential for quality of life. Money can solve many problems, but it means very little if you are in poor health. Trying to get rich at the expense of one's wellbeing is not smart. You cannot enjoy the financial fruits of your labour if you're in constant pain, unable to move, struggling to breathe, going to the hospital every few months, or worrying about your health.

To that end, my daily routine is important to me. Most mornings I am up at 4am and in the gym at 5am doing cardio or lifting weights and giving my central nervous system an absolute blast to fire me up for the day. Then it's off to do a full day's work at 7am. Most evenings, I do some yoga to relax and slow down my central nervous system and get ready for a good night's sleep. Rinse and repeat the next day. I also take part in weekly local five-kilometre park runs and various ten-kilometre running festivals in Melbourne.

Pat and I also enjoy plenty of healthy pursuits together – cooking healthy foods and going to the gym, yoga classes (my handstand and downward dog are looking pretty good, I must say) and health retreats. Oh, and giving up the booze (mostly) has probably helped too.

We intend to make the most of every moment we have together, for as long as we have together: '… for better, for worse, for richer, for poorer, in sickness and in health, to love and to cherish, 'til death do us part.'

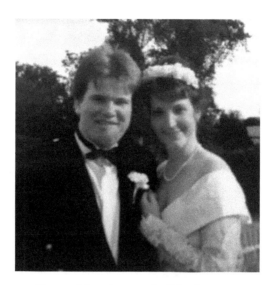

The wedding that nearly didn't happen.

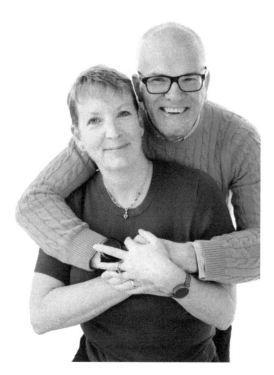

Here and now – living our best life.

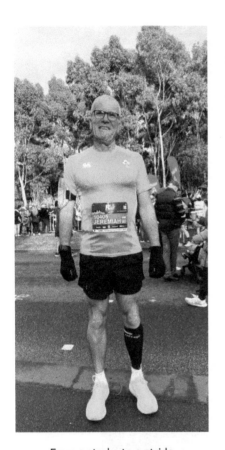

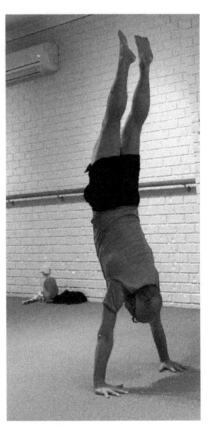

From a stroke to a stride
– Melbourne 10 km.

Upside down and loving
life Down Under.

The Things You Can Control

Navigating through trauma, whether from the domestic violence I witnessed or the severe health challenges I faced, feels like being imprisoned in an inescapable cell. It can mentally paralyse and utterly overwhelm you, making simple tasks like getting out of bed or going to work seem insurmountable. Trauma wields the power to consume your entire existence, casting a heavy shadow over every aspect of your life.

My mind would incessantly replay my childhood experiences of domestic violence without ever finding closure. The fear and anxiety only intensified, spiralling into a torrent of negative emotions trapped in an endless cycle. Not only did my thoughts dwell on past events but they also exaggerated potential scenarios, leading to heightened stress. My mind grappled with understanding why bad things kept happening and how they might worsen further.

Even years after my operation, terrifying nightmares of bleeding to death haunted me relentlessly. Every night, I relived the horror of my teeth falling out amid a deluge of blood pouring from my mouth. The sheer terror would jolt me awake, screaming and babbling incoherently, my mind still trapped in the gruesome scenes. Pat, with endless patience, would comfort me, trying to bring me back to reality. Only when I fully grasped that I was safe at home did the panic subside, allowing me to finally relax and find solace in my surroundings.

So how did I rise above it? I survived the trauma and learned to cope with my escalating emotions. It started with transforming my negative thoughts into positive ones, recognising the importance of cultivating habits that foster positive actions for both mind and body. I learned to accept all feelings that enter my mind, acknowledging their transience; they won't last forever. Letting go of the past became crucial (even though I did try to invent a time machine for my third-year university project, it's simply impossible).

Embracing the present became my guiding principle, leading me to divide it into two distinct categories:

1. The immediate present (the here and now, focusing on the next few minutes and hours): I centre myself by concentrating on my breath – inhaling for four seconds, holding for two, and exhaling slowly for six seconds. This simple yet powerful breathing technique became my anchor during near-death experiences, helping me regulate my heart rate and mitigate blood loss.

2. The near present (looking to the days and weeks ahead): I made a conscious effort to stop fixating on hypothetical futures that may never materialise. While it's important to consider all options and prepare contingency plans (I am a project manager after all), dwelling excessively on negatives only fuels a cycle of negativity. I realised the immense influence our thoughts and words wield. As a result, I know it's imperative to envision success rather than anticipate failure.

I also redirected the energy and time spent on negative thoughts by changing my internal dialogue. When faced with a challenge, instead of saying to myself, 'I can't,' I would ask myself, 'What can I do?' After my stroke, when I was paralysed on my right side, I could have easily given up because I could not walk. Instead, I asked myself, 'What can I do?' I could walk with a walking frame, taking small steps and making incremental improvements that ultimately led me not only to walk but to run again.

In essence, I've come to realise there are only two things I can really control in my life: my thoughts and my actions. It was imperative for me to escape from the treacherous downward spiral of negative thinking that pushed me to want to kill myself. I had to make that choice and commit to it. Similarly, my actions are within my domain of control. I cannot dictate other people's thoughts, words or actions towards me, but I wield the power to choose how I respond. This involves embracing life's challenges with resilience and perseverance, and accepting reality as it is rather than clinging to any illusions of what I wish it to be. I've learned to have a sense of perspective.

I think back to that time post-operation when I was paralysed in a hospital bed, unable to eat, drink, speak or move. I was shitting the bed and being turned every two hours to prevent pressure sores. Nothing can compare to that suffering, and it serves as a constant reminder that life is too short to hold back and dwell on trivial matters. It's too valuable to squander on negativity.

In the grand scheme of things, the universe doesn't really care if I am happy or sad. The sun will still rise and set as it has done for the last five billion years (and will do for another five billion years). An average human, therefore, only lives for 0.00000075 per cent of the sun's life. In this cosmic context, our human life span is insignificant. This knowledge has humbled me and has taught me to find happiness and gratitude in the simplicity of life.

My greatest battles have been waged in my own mind, and it has taken me years to become comfortable in my own skin. So I would say to you, if you have read this far: never, ever give up. You can get through the dark days. My story is proof positive you can survive – and learn to thrive.

Acknowledgements

To George for being the father I never had. What a guy you are. You took on all the baggage of a single mum with two young children and raised them as your own. To this day you are still there by my mother's side as she suffers and slowly deteriorates from the 'long goodbye' – dementia.

To my sister, Sharon, her husband, Emmet, and their daughter, Kirsten, for always having my back and always being there.

To my brother, Paul – you missed your childhood because I spent so much time in hospital, with Mum and George there to support me through my medical dramas. The focus was always on me – for this, I am truly sorry.

To the unknown dental student who was brave enough to speak up and tell his superior, 'I think we have a problem here. We should not take that tooth out.' If it wasn't for you, I would have bled to death and I would not be writing this story.

To John Anthony Lynn, consultant vascular surgeon. You established an international reputation in your field and took on the most complicated of vascular operations – high-flow AVMs like mine.

To the director of diagnostic radiology at the Hammersmith Hospital, Professor David John Allison – a pioneer in developing the embolisation procedure on the most complicated of AVMs. You are an absolute legend both professionally and personally. Every radiologist in the world has probably read *Diagnostic Radiology: An Anglo-American Textbook of Imaging*, simply known as 'Grainger and Allison'. The first radiologist in the UK to embolise pulmonary arteriovenous malformations, in the early 1980s, you had the foresight to start building the first fully digital hospital in the world. In addition to your extraordinary clinical outputs, I will be forever grateful to you for saving my life on so many occasions by carrying out emergency embolisations, as otherwise I would certainly have bled to death.

To James Jackson, consultant radiologist, who took over from Professor Allison at the Hammersmith Hospital. Apart from Professor Allison, you were the only other radiologist I trusted to carry out embolisations on my face. High-flow AVMs like mine require the best of the best. You are the best – clinical excellence personified.

To Colin Hopper, the maxillofacial surgeon, who held my mandible together during the operation. Over the years after the operation, you were always available when I had any issues.

To Per Hall, the plastic surgeon, who is not only a fantastic surgeon but a great human.

To Ali Hudson, for saving my life that night as we flew by helicopter to the Hammersmith Hospital. You nearly lost your job in the process because you left the ward unattended.

To Liz, the physio, and Sue, the speech therapist, who both got me on the road to recovery as I learned to talk, walk and eat all over again.

To Father Richard Arrandale for making the wedding happen. Without you, Pat and I would not be married. May you rest in peace: 27 June 2008.

To all my family and friends – from the early days in the Drum at St Pius primary and secondary schools, through university and throughout my career. I thank you for helping me be the person I am today. I am privileged to have known so many good humans with such kind hearts and good souls.

To all my personal trainers who have helped me achieve and exceed my fitness goals in the gym: Lynda Wilson, Troy Reneker, Alana Lynch, Kelly-Anne Southgate, Jody Mielke, Renee Hinks, Rachelle Cain and Daryl Segrave (aka Big Bad Daz).

To all my yoga teachers: Mary Rollo, Leesa Patten and Bec Caldwell for helping me develop my breath and strength of mind and body. And in particular Michelle Caldwell at Yoga 101 for your patience, commitment and focus on ensuring I get the best out of my body, and maintaining and improving my flexibility, balance, mental clarity and concentration – and also for catching me when I fall over doing handstands.

To Heather Millar who helped me write this story. At times I struggled to articulate on some difficult topics and you probed, questioned and challenged me to truly express how I felt. For this, I thank you.

The final words of acknowledgement must go to the two most important humans in my life who have shown me complete and total unconditional love – my mother and Pat.

To my mother who carried me for nine months, protected me from Big Jerry when I was scared and lonely as a child, who stood by my bedside as I lay bleeding, close to death on a number of occasions. I can't imagine the shock you would have felt when you received a call from the hospital saying, 'Jerry is bleeding to death and you need to get to the hospital quickly before he dies' – and then on your arrival you meet the priest leaving my bedside after he has just given me the last rites. Your sacrifice, your selflessness and your compassion know no boundaries. The reason I know how to love and be loved is because of you. I love you and I miss you.

To Pat – since the first day we met in hospital (even when I couldn't see you), I felt a connection. I could never really explain it. I never believed in fate – but I have often thought that if I had not gone through the physical and mental pain I endured, I would not have met you. I had nothing to offer you – I was a physical and mental wreck. I was close to death and with an uncertain future and yet you saw something in me that I couldn't see within myself. They said our marriage wouldn't last. Remember that time we were refused a house mortgage because the bank said I would die before the mortgage would be paid off? I was too much of a risk. We have shown that no matter what comes our way in life, good or bad, we will only be parted by death. Until that day, we share our love unconditionally as we continue this journey on planet Earth as two souls that have been and always will be intertwined physically, mentally and spiritually.

Printed in Australia
Ingram Content Group Australia Pty Ltd
AUHW011204310724
397779AU00010B/117